Evidence-based Pharmacy

Evidence-based Pharmacy

Edited by

Christine Bond

BPharm, MEd, PhD, MRPharmS

Senior Lecturer and Deputy Head of Department
Department of General Practice and Primary Care
University of Aberdeen
Aberdeen, UK

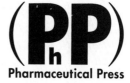

Pharmaceutical Press

Published by the Pharmaceutical Press

An imprint of RPS Publishing

1 Lambeth High Street, London SE1 7JN, UK

100 South Atkinson Road, Suite 200, Grayslake, IL 60030-7820, USA

© Pharmaceutical Press 2000

$\left(\mathbf{PP}\right)$ is a trade mark of RPS Publishing

RPS Publishing is the publishing organisation of the Royal
Pharmaceutical Society of Great Britain

First published 2000
Reprinted 2001, 2002, 2003, 2006, 2009

Text design by Barker/Hilsdon, Lyme Regis, Dorset
Typeset by Type Study, Scarborough, North Yorkshire
Printed in Great Britain by TJ International, Padstow, Cornwall

ISBN 978 0 85369 436 6

A catalogue record for this book is available from the British Library.

For Chris, Philip, Simon and Niall

Contents

Foreword

We have been talking about evidence-based pharmacy for many years. The Royal Pharmaceutical Society's *pharmacy in a new age* initiative and, more recently, the advent of clinical governance have emphasised that now is the time to turn all that talk into action. Here is a book, looking at the key target areas of *building the future*, that will point us in the right direction! This is the place to start for researchers and pharmacists working in primary care. It will enable us to raise awareness of the available research and to define what still needs to be done.

As a profession we may understand our worth, but how do we convince others?

It is becoming increasingly important to gather the evidence to support our claims for the usefulness and quality of service that we can provide. Such evidence will be vital at a national level as the Society and others seek to convince the government and professional bodies of the pharmacist's value. At a local level, where responsibility for service commissioning and funding is being increasingly devolved, pharmacists will need evidence to support their arguments to deliver a range of new services.

The Society fully supports the need to get research into pharmacy practice and is taking steps to make this happen. Pharmacy Development Groups (PDGs) are forming in England and Wales, and locality groups in Scotland, with membership across the profession, looking at ways of taking the profession forward in their localities. PDGs will be linked by pdgtalk.net, a closed internet discussion group, to help spread ideas and best practice.

Professional development awards have been made available, through a bidding process, to help groups develop their infrastructure and to take forward their initiatives. Practice research will be crucial to support a PDG's work, and I hope PDGs themselves will take up the challenge, undertaking and disseminating their own research.

I have no doubt that the authors of this book would be the first to acknowledge that more work needs to be done in this field. I hope that many of you will take up the themes within these pages to help *build the future* for generations of pharmacists to come.

Christine Glover
President, Royal Pharmaceutical Society of Great Britain
March 2000

Preface

This book has been produced for two reasons. It is intended to highlight some of the new services pharmacists are providing in the community, to give the background to these services and provide research evidence to demonstrate their benefit. Thus we can claim that the new age for pharmacy is built not only on the consensus of the profession and its vision of the future, but also on evidence-based practice; i.e. it is in the true spirit of the clinical effectiveness and clinical governance agenda. Thus this book should be of value to those wishing to implement the services described, perhaps in their Primary Care Groups, where other professional colleagues may not be familiar with the body of literature and evidence which can demonstrate the added value a pharmacist can make to patient care.

Secondly, because pharmacy practice research is still a fledgling discipline in academic terms, there are few books available which can illustrate the health services research methodologies used in pharmacy practice research with examples from pharmacy. This book will, I hope, do that, and should therefore be of interest to pharmacy practice researchers developing projects at undergraduate and at postgraduate levels. There is also a need for all pharmacists to be research aware, and to be able to critically discuss research findings, before deciding whether the results reported are justified, and should be disseminated and used. Thus all pharmacists should find this book of use as studies are reported and discussed critically by the respective chapter authors, in much the same way as a good research paper or research thesis should highlight problems and confounders and interpret results accordingly. Whilst each chapter has been written so that it can be read for detailed information on specific topics, more will be gained if the book is read sequentially as presented.

The book is structured so that the history of pharmacy practice research and the theoretical justification for research evidence is presented in the preliminary chapter, followed by individual chapters which address one aspect of the Pharmacy in a New Age themes. As shown in the final chapter the only theme not directly covered is 'advice to other health professionals'. However, there is overlap between this and most of the topics covered. Each chapter is structured to give an introduction to the topic, the research question, an example or examples of relevant studies, and the implications for future practice. In this way, different methodologies are introduced to the reader through relevant examples. As practice develops, and with the luxury of hindsight, these may not necessarily be the topics we would choose to research today, and the methods we might choose would be refined in the light of new methodologies. However, at this point in time, I think the studies presented have all been milestones in the development of both practice research and professional development. In the closing chapter, the extent and robustness of the evidence presented is considered.

I am very grateful to the author of each chapter for giving of their time to contribute to this book and for sharing their thoughts on the future. I believe that they have given us an excellent foundation on which to build.

Christine Bond
Aberdeen, April 2000

About the editor

Dr Bond has worked for Glaxo Research Laboratories, has had extensive locum community pharmacist experience and is now Senior Lecturer and Deputy Head of Department in the Department of General
Practice and Primary Care, University of Aberdeen. She is Head of
Undergraduate General Practice teaching and has an extensive research
portfolio, with over 100 publications. Her main research interests are in
the pharmacist's role in the optimum use of medicines, both prescribed
and over the counter, and the contribution of community pharmacy to
the wider primary healthcare agenda. She is currently seconded to
Grampian Health Board as a part-time Consultant in Pharmaceutical
Public Health (CAPO), and is a member of the Royal Pharmaceutical
Society of Great Britain Scottish Executive.

Contributors

Alison Blenkinsopp PhD, MRPharmS
Professor of the Practice of Pharmacy
Department of Medicines Management
Keele University
Keele, Staffordshire, UK

Christine Bond PhD, MEd, MRPharmS
Senior Lecturer
Department of General Practice and Primary Care
University of Aberdeen
Aberdeen, UK

Sheena Macgregor MRPharmS
Senior Prescribing Adviser
Borders Primary Care Trust
Newstead, Melrose, Roxburghshire

Catriona Matheson PhD, MRPharmS
Research Fellow
Department of General Practice and Primary Care
University of Aberdeen
Aberdeen, UK

Mandy Ryan PhD
MRC Senior Fellow and Health Economist
Health Economic Research Unit
University of Aberdeen
Aberdeen, UK

Hazel Sinclair PhD
Research Fellow
Department of General Practice and Primary Care
University of Aberdeen
Aberdeen, UK

Felicity Smith PhD, MRPharmS
Senior Lecturer
School of Pharmacy
University of London
London, UK

Sharon Williams PhD, MRPharmS
Research Fellow
Department of General Practice and Primary Care
University of Aberdeen
Aberdeen, UK

1

An introduction to pharmacy practice research

Christine Bond

Introduction

The purpose of this book is to consider the changing practice of community pharmacy, and to consider the place of research in driving and informing that process. Research uses standard methods to describe events in an objective way, to minimise the misrepresentation of facts and to allow generalisation of findings from the sample studied to the wider population. Research may be descriptive, to provide an accurate picture of current practice, or it may be empirical, and identify causal associations between new practice and observed results on the basis of experimental interventions. Methods may be quantitative or qualitative, and in many studies both types of method will be used to inform the other. Thus a quantitative questionnaire may be informed by qualitative in-depth content-setting focus group discussions to ensure key issues are covered.

A new age for pharmacy

In the past pharmacists have been referred to as over-trained for what they do and under-utilised in what they know (Eaton and Webb, 1979). This is said to be in comparison with the status of the profession in other countries, for example France, where pharmacy has developed as one of the great professions (Trease, 1965). There is clear evidence that the status of the profession in the hospital context has increased since the parallel increase in its clinical role (Smith and Knapp, 1972; Cotter *et al.*, 1994). There is now an awareness at a national, multi-disciplinary, level that there should be an equivalent increased utilisation of the community pharmacist, although restricted access to the prescriber (Barber *et al.*, 1994), may result in different models of care developing, compared to the hospital setting. Exactly how this might be done and an exploration of some of the wider issues are the basis for this book, in which selected key issues are researched to provide an evidence base for their future implementation into practice.

Recognition that the profession of pharmacy was no longer being utilised to its full potential, due to external factors, was first officially identified in 1979 by the Royal Commission on the NHS (Merrison, 1979) and described in other subsequent reports as detailed in Table 1.1.

Extensive consultation both within and outside the profession resulted in the most definitive description of the future role of community

Table 1.1 The major reports considering future role of pharmacy (Bond 1999)[a]

Date	Report	Remit
1979	Report on the NHS (HMSO)	The best use and management of the financial and manpower resources of the NHS.
1986	Pharmacy: a report to the Nuffield Foundation	Consideration of the present and future structure of pharmacy, its contribution to healthcare, its education and training.
1987	Promoting Better Health (HMSO)	Proposals to improve primary healthcare and the services offered to patients.
1989	Role and Function of the pharmacist in Europe (WHO)	A definition of the functions and responsibilities of the pharmacist in the healthcare system of an industrialised country and recommendations for further development.
1989	Working for patients (HMSO)	Proposals to give patients better health-care and greater choice of services; to give greater satisfaction and rewards for those working in the NHS who respond to local needs.
1992	Pharmaceutical Care: the future for community pharmacy (DoH)	Consideration of ways in which the NHS community pharmaceutical services might be developed to increase their contribution to healthcare and to make recommendations.
1992	Community pharmacies in England (NAO)	The economy, efficiency and effectiveness of community pharmacy.
1997	Primary Care: Agenda for Action	A coherent development programme for primary care in Scotland, with specific references to community pharmacy throughout, with reference in particular to developing capacity and improving service delivery.

[a]Based on a table first published in Primary Health Care Sciences, 1999, London: Whurr.

pharmacy: 'Pharmaceutical Care: the future for community pharmacy' (Department of Health, 1992) produced jointly by the Department of Health and the Royal Pharmaceutical Society of Great Britain. This document considered various aspects of the community pharmacist's working practice under nine broad headings, including services to general practitioners, the over-the-counter (OTC) advisory role, health promotion, and services to special needs groups such as the housebound. Thirty specific tasks were listed in the annex, which were recommended for introduction nationally or on a pilot basis. Whilst some of these tasks merely formalised ongoing practice and were generally welcomed, others were innovative, covering areas as diverse as simple healthcare advice to therapeutic drug monitoring, and prescribing following agreed protocols. The report was received with some reservations by medical bodies (Anonymous, 1992a) and welcomed as 'pragmatic, prosaic, and progressive' by the pharmaceutical profession (Anonymous, 1992b; Anonymous, 1992c).

More recently, the profession itself has undertaken a profession-wide consultation process to consider the future. This has been called, successively, the 'New Age for Pharmacy', the 'New Horizon', and 'Building the Future'. The programme, now known as PIANA (Pharmacy in a New Age) has drawn on pharmacy practice research and evaluated examples of good practice to inform its debate. Some of the key studies contribute to this book.

Finally, the reality of the extended role has been aided by an overall review of healthcare by central government in 1997. The White Papers from England (Department of Health, 1997), Wales (Secretary of State for Wales, 1998), and Scotland (Secretary of State for Scotland, 1997), all identify opportunities for pharmacy in relation to medicines management, clinical effectiveness, and clinical governance. Although the profession per se is not often mentioned specifically, the roles are clearly spelt out. Pharmacy's justification to deliver new roles will be enhanced by robust studies which provide evidence not only for the ability of the profession to carry out a role, but also for its ability to carry it out as well as, or better than, other professions. This is an exciting time for the profession, with new opportunities for the professional base of pharmacy to expand again; this is more likely to become a reality if supported by evidence.

A key feature in the changing practice of pharmacy is the pivotal place of drug utilisation and medicines management as an area of professional responsibility. These are subjects for which community pharmacists are uniquely qualified and this is exemplified by the advice which is given to both general medical practitioners and the public. In the context of an ever-increasing emphasis on clinically effective and cost effective use of medicines, both of these roles are currently expanding, with an increase in the numbers of pharmacists working in general medical practices and with the increased number of potent drugs available for over-the-counter (OTC) sale from community pharmacies. Both of these topics are the subject of individual chapters in this book.

Pharmacy practice research and health services research

Historical aspects

Pharmacy practice research is a relatively new discipline. It has been defined by the Pharmacy Practice Research Task Force (1997) as:

> research which attempts to inform and understand pharmacy and the way in which it is practiced, in order to ensure that pharmacists' knowledge and skills are used to the best effect in solving the problems of the health service and meeting the needs of the population and to support the objectives of pharmacy practice.

It is in many ways a branch of health services research, another relatively new discipline which is 'the investigation of the health needs of the community and the effectiveness and efficiency of the provision of services to meet those needs' (Medical Research Council, 1993). However, pharmacy practice research looks specifically at pharmacy-related events, and the pharmaceutical interface with other professions and the public. It does, however, utilise many of the methodologies developed by health service researchers for use in the study of the provision of healthcare. Many of these have been adopted from consumer research in other contexts.

Both health services research and pharmacy practice research are expanding disciplines, required at a time of change in the NHS, to inform new practice and provide information on the cost effectiveness and efficiency of different service delivery options. In order to support pharmacy practice research and to provide an infrastructure within the profession, the Pharmacy Enterprise Scheme was launched in England and Wales in April 1990 and was funded until the end of the financial year 1997/98. The purpose of the scheme was to train a new generation of pharmacy practice researchers through sponsored higher degrees, either research-based and leading to masters or doctorates, or taught masters. This was done through a combination of studentships, training awards and project development grants. Successful applicants were largely based in academic departments other than pharmacy, such as health economic units, departments of general practice, sociology, and psychology. In total, 91 awards were made (21 PhD studentships, 32 training awards and 38 project development grants). Full details of the achievements of the scheme are published in their Resource Document (Pharmacy Practice Research Resource Centre, 1997).

In Scotland, pharmacists were not eligible for the enterprise scheme, but equivalent resources were allocated to a pharmacy practice research fund, to which individual researchers applied on a competitive, annual basis for funding for specific projects. In this way a range of projects have been funded, and some of these are reported in Chapters 3 and 6 of this book.

One of the first formal acknowledgements by the profession of pharmacy practice research was the introduction of a practice research session at the annual British Pharmaceutical Conference. The first session was in 1977. In recent years, the practice research 'session' has increased to several sessions of oral presentations plus a large poster display, and this is beginning to match the contributions of the basic sciences. Because the format of the abstracts for these presentations is that of a mini-paper, and because they are published as a supplement to the *Pharmaceutical Journal* each year, perusal of this series of supplements provides a useful profile of the progress within practice research to date.

The first dedicated practice research conference was held in 1991 at the Royal Pharmaceutical Society's headquarters in Lambeth, London (Pharmacy Practice Research Conference Proceedings, 1991). At this conference the establishment of a Pharmacy Practice Research Resource Centre, as part of the Enterprise Scheme, was announced, to be supported by the Department of Health for a fixed period of five years. After a consultation period, the centre was established within the Pharmacy Department at the University of Manchester, but with an independent board of management, and under the inaugural leadership of Professor Peter Noyce. The centre existed to stimulate and support research and development activities amongst practising community pharmacists. The centre has been instrumental in promoting and supporting pharmacy practice research through a range of initiatives. One of the most effective of these is its series of briefing papers on research methods, which, as a complete collection, provides an excellent introduction to the range of research methodologies required to carry out research in this field.

The papers are also extensively referenced for those wishing for more detailed information.

There have been two other pivotal activities from the Pharmacy Practice Research Resource Centre, which have been central to the development of the discipline. First, the centre has commissioned, as part of its portfolio of activities, a series of occasional papers. The third document in the series was a review of pharmacy practice research to date. Commissioned from Nicholas Mays, then Director of Health and Health Care Research Unit at the Queen's University Belfast, subsequently Director of Health Services Research at the King's Fund Institute and most recently Adviser to the Health Social Policy Branch of the New Zealand Treasury, the review provided the focus for a conference on health services research and pharmacy, held in London in 1994.

This review was commissioned to provide an external assessment of the current state of the discipline, from a respected health services researcher. The review concluded that, at that time, the discipline was immature and limited to small descriptive and feasibility studies, largely conducted by pharmacists with an apparent objective of proving that an individual pharmacist could provide almost any service. Whilst studies such as these have a place as feasibility exercises, in the context of health services it is essential to move onto the stage of exploring what the profession as a whole can deliver (not just highly trained, motivated or dedicated individuals) and the relative costs and benefits of a service being provided by the pharmacy profession in comparison to other healthcare professionals, e.g. nursing or medical colleagues. This report also indicated the need, therefore, to include in pharmacy practice research disciplines other than pharmacy, such as behavioural scientists, sociologists, psychologists, anthropologists and health economists.

The other pivotal action of the Centre was the establishment of a new annual Pharmacy Practice Research and Health Services Research Conference to provide a forum for presenting results and methodological issues. The first conference was held in Birmingham in 1995 and has now become a well-supported annual event. Finally, another forum for disseminating pharmacy practice research on the international scene is the Social Pharmacy Conference, which has provided a biennial opportunity for researchers to meet and exchange ideas since 1978.

Soon after the review of practice research authored by Nicholas Mays, the Royal Pharmaceutical Society of Great Britain appointed Dr Sue Ambler to the post of Head of Practice Research with a remit to develop pharmacy practice research. She established a multidisciplinary task force to review the state of pharmacy practice and make recommendations for the future. The task force was chaired by Nicholas Mays and although comprising a large number of pharmacists with a range of backgrounds, also included representatives of nursing, medicine, the pharmaceutical industry and sociology.

Pharmacy practice has been defined by the task force as:

> The application of the knowledge and skills of pharmacists, and the infra-structure of pharmacy, to meeting the health needs of the population. This should be performed in a manner which is equitable, effective, efficient, appropriate, acceptable and relevant, and which is attainable in the commercial and other contexts in which pharmacy is practiced.

The task force reported back to invited representatives of the profession in 1997 at a meeting held, again, at the King's Fund in London. Their conclusions were also published as a full report (Royal Pharmaceutical Society of Great Britain, 1997a) and as a briefing paper (Royal Pharmaceutical Society of Great Britain, 1997b). The task force believed that the research agenda must:

- identify critical questions, research issues and priorities of the health service, major funding bodies and investors in pharmacy practice research;
- place the pharmacy research questions in a wider health and social care context;
- take into account and reflect issues of interest to all key stakeholders in pharmacy;
- take a balanced view of all appropriate research perspectives, approaches and conceptual frameworks in prioritising the research questions;
- generate rigorous, reproducible and generalisable results which can be applied on a national basis;
- take full account of the commercial context in which pharmacy is often practised.

Since the task force reported back, there has been a final stage in the agenda setting for practice research. This is being done through a systematic consensus procedure, once again co-ordinated by the Pharmacy Practice Research Resource Centre. Under three main themes of Self-care and Pharmacy, Drug Therapy and Pharmacy, and Workforce Issues, multidisciplinary expert groups have been convened, first, to consider specially commissioned briefing papers, and then to propose a research agenda, which has been refined after consultation with invited representatives of different branches of the profession. The final reports of the first two of these three initiatives are available from the Royal Pharmaceutical Society of Great Britain.

Once again, Scotland was not totally integrated into this approach to setting the research agenda, although individual practitioners from Scotland have been consulted for their particular expertise. It is only relatively recently, in 1998, that a Scottish Practice Research Fellow has been appointed to move forward the agenda in Scotland. However, not withstanding this, many practice research studies have been carried out to date in Scotland, and have greatly influenced the extended professional practice that is now accepted as the norm.

Evidence-based practice

The Cochrane Collaboration was established in 1993 (Dickersin and Manheimer, 1998) as a result of a meeting of minds. It is a worldwide multidisciplinary network of individuals with a commitment to evidence-based healthcare, and grew out of a realisation that much clinical practice did not reflect the most recent research; that much research which was published was not necessarily of the highest quality; that practitioners were unable to find the time either to read all the relevant journals in order to keep up to date or to review the evidence critically; and that, using a technique called meta-analysis, it was possible to pool the results of many small, albeit robust, studies to get virtual large studies with increased statistical power and discrimination.

One of the most significant achievements of the Cochrane Collaboration, apart from the amassing of a lot of very relevant evidence-based systematic reviews, is increased awareness of the necessity of looking critically at the methodology of a study before any of the actual results are considered. If the method is flawed, then the study may as well not have been conducted and the research is of little or no value. In order to help quickly identify what are known as the 'right sort of studies' – that is, those of a sufficiently high standard to justify considering the results – levels or grades of evidence have been defined. These are as follows:

- Level 1 A randomised control trial (RCT).
- Level 2 A case controlled trial.
- Level 3 A controlled before and after study.
- Level 4 Observational data.

With each type of method, there are checklists to ensure that the study truly fulfils the methodological requirements. Thus, for a randomised

controlled trial there needs to be information within the paper confirming, for example, that the randomisation was done to the approved
methods, that there was no opportunity for contamination between the
groups, that assessors were blind to group membership and that the right
statistical tests were used.

The Collaboration has sub-groups called editorial groups with
their own management structures. The one most relevant to pharmacy
practice is EPOC (Effective Practice and Organization of Care), formerly
known as CCEPP (Cochrane Collaboration for Effective Professional
Practice) and was established in 1995. Anyone with an interest can register a topic, for example the effect of expanding pharmacists' roles (Bero
et al., 1997), and submit a protocol for a systematic review of the topic.
This is reviewed by the Editorial Board and, if it meets the standards,
the group will carry out a search for all the relevant studies, which are
then combined into an overall review and conclusion. In the case of the
Bero review on expanding pharmacists' roles, it was concluded, on the
basis of 12 identified randomised controlled trials, that pharmacist
management of drug therapy can successfully substitute for patient
management by physicians; education of physicians by pharmacists is
not as successful as education of physicians by other physicians; and that
delivery of services by pharmacists decreases the use and/or costs of
health services and improves patient outcomes compared to no comparable service. The review concludes that the implications for practice
are therefore that pharmacists should continue their roles in delivering
patient counselling regarding drug therapy, and educating physicians
about drug therapy. The implications for research are whether better or
comparable services can be delivered by pharmacists at lower cost compared to physicians, and to ensure that patient outcome measures should
always include assessments of adverse drug events and quality of life.

Following on from Cochrane, there has a been a move in Scotland
to use systematic search techniques combined with professional input to
draw up evidence-based guidelines for best treatments. This movement,
known as SIGN (Scottish Intercollegiate Network), has the support of
the Royal Medical Colleges, and to date has drawn up over 40 guidelines on topics such as primary prevention of cardiovascular disease,
Helicobacter pylori eradication, etc. Most of the review teams have
pharmacy input.

SIGN has acknowledged that there may be instances where evidence from an RCT does not exist and that lesser levels of evidence may
have to be used if this is the best available. Indeed, it has also been said
that RCTs and evidence-based medicine are not necessarily always the

most appropriate (Anonymous, 1998) both because of the art of medicine, clinical judgement and patient variability, and because a RCT not conducted to the best standards, or not measuring the most relevant outcomes, will not be the gold standard that we seek. In addition, as clearly defended recently by Green and Britten (1998), qualitative research methods can help bridge the gap between scientific practice and clinical practice. Qualitative findings can provide rigorous accounts of treatment regimes in everyday practice, which can help us understand the barriers to using evidence-based medicine, and its limitations. This allows us to understand that some research questions require different types of research to answer them.

Methods in health services research

As indicated earlier, the types of research methodology used in practice research owe more to a heritage from market research than the laboratory traditions of the pharmaceutical sciences. A summary of the main types of research and their strengths and weaknesses are shown in Table 1.2, together with a reference to the chapter in which this type of research is used.

In the remainder of this section, a brief description of some of these key methodologies is presented. Further details will also be found in the individual topic chapters.

Questionnaire surveys

Questionnaire surveys are widely used in many practice research studies to provide descriptive information on total populations and/or large representative random samples of pharmacists, general practitioners and the public. Much of the original pharmacy practice research uses surveys to assess levels of current practice and quantify attitudes (Mays, 1994).

The basic principles of questionnaire design should always be followed as defined by standard texts (Oppenheim, 1993; Moser and Kalton, 1993). In outline, questions should be selected after extensive literature review of the relevant field, with additional content setting information obtained from, for example, focus group discussions or consultation with topic experts and individual users. The wording of questions must be carefully scrutinised by the researcher to avoid ambiguity, imprecision, double questions, double negatives, inappropriate vocabulary, and leading or presumptive questions. Questions seeking retrospective information should be kept to a minimum because of the reduced accuracy of such data. Structured answer formats aid analysis, such as yes/no types, lists, categories, scaling, quantity and grid. In general, structured questions should additionally provide an 'other' or 'don't know' facility. Some open questions may need to be included where a structured format could not cover all the possibilities; and these can either be coded as a discrete exercise or at the point of data entry. Questionnaire length and layout must be considered in the context of maximising response rate; that is, questionnaires must be produced to a high standard, so that the appearance is attractive and user-friendly. Questions should be sequenced in as logical and interesting a way as possible, whilst avoiding any 'leading' effect. Easier questions should be at the beginning and sensitive or more difficult questions at the end. Precautions must be taken to ensure that the ordering of questions does not affect the nature of the response, and in some instances, the questions or attitude statements should be randomised using random number tables. Options for completion of individual questions must be made clear. Initially, draft questionnaires should be prepared and pre-piloted on small groups of selected individuals, followed where possible by piloting on a random sample of the population to be studied, having already identified and then excluded the study sample. Comments should be invited from the pre-pilot responders on relevance of questions as well as checking for other flaws. Results from the formal pilot will further confirm these points. In the pilot, likely response rates can be assessed and results scrutinised and/or analysed to ensure that the questionnaire is correctly identifying the key issues.

Samples for questionnaire surveys should always be randomly selected, unless the total population in question is being surveyed. Sometimes random number tables may be used to identify a sample from an agreed sampling frame or sequential sampling may be used. Sometimes prior stratification of the population may be required to ensure equal distribution of factors perceived likely to affect the responses, and quota sampling may be used to ensure that minority groups are included.

Two-phase sampling (the simplest form of multiphase sampling) can be used if asking all the sample to collect the detailed information required is likely to jeopardise response rates. Thus the most important information required is included in an initial questionnaire to the whole sample. More detailed, or time-consuming elements for completion, for example, prospective information collected through completion of a daily log over a week-long period, is then only collected by a self-selected sub-sample and the consequent limitations of this are acknowledged.

Questionnaires are most usually distributed by post, and should

Table 1.2 A summary of research methods

Research method	Application	Chapter reference	Control	Strengths	Weaknesses
Survey	Perceived value of guidelines	3	None	Representative of population	Only cross sectional data Validity of questionnaire Response rates
	Services provided to drug misusers by community pharmacists	9			
	Attitudes to drug misusers	9			
	Attitudes of GPs to deregulated medicines	3			
Experimental 1	Value of guidelines in improving knowledge	3	Group acted as own control with unrelated guideline questions	High validity Good control	Artificial: effect on patient outcome unknown
	Disease management	6			
Experimental 2 (RCT)	Prescribing 1	5	Controls	High validity	
	Smoking cessation	8			
Field research: Case study	Development of guidelines	3	None	Study events in natural setting	Ethical considerations of participant observation Subjective data collection and evaluation

Table 1.2 continued

Research method	Application	Chapter reference	Control	Strengths	Weaknesses
Field research: Observation	Development of guidelines Advice giving role Drug misuse	3 2 9	None	Study events in natural setting	Subjective Researcher may influence events ('Hawthorne effect')
Field research Interviews	Opinions of community pharmacists (smoking cessation, drug misuse)	8, 9	None	Can develop issues as they arise Good response rate	Interviewer may influence responses
Existing data research	Economic modelling	4	None	Data not influenced by researcher	Data not always in correct format Retrospective

include a reply-paid or stamped envelope or 'Freepost' address for return of the completed questionnaire. Reminders should be sent approximately three and six weeks after the original mailing, and include replacement questionnaires. Sometimes respondents can be reminded by telephone if response rates are poor. All questionnaires should be totally confidential, identifiable by a unique code purely for the purpose of following up non-responders. Data stored should comply with the requirements of the Data Protection Act. Where total anonymity is necessary because of the sensitive nature of the questions, a method developed by Taylor (1992) and first used in 1986 (Taylor *et al.*, 1986) can be used which still allows identification and follow-up of non-responders. In this method, at the same time as the uniden-tified questionnaire is returned by the respondent, an identifiable reply-paid postcard is also mailed confirming that the completed ques-tionnaire has been posted. Experience shows that the returns match up numerically.

The importance of a good response rate cannot be overstated, as poor response rates may lead to serious bias. Moser and Kalton (1993) state that:

> a poor response rate must constitute a dangerous failing and if it does not rise above, say 20 or 30% the failing is so critical as to make the survey results of little, if any, value.

Other texts (Pharmacy Practice Research Resource Centre, 1992) have recommended a minimum response rate of 66%. This higher response rate seems to me to be necessary, because even at 70%, should all the non-responders hold an opposite view to the majority of the responders, the conclusions of the survey could be totally reversed. Wherever poss-ible, any information on non-responders must be analysed to allow identification of any data that are obviously unrepresentative.

Telephone interviews

Telephone interviews can be useful to provide more in-depth qualitative information on a small sample of the population as in interviewing generally (see later) or for completion of a structured questionnaire to maximise response rate. This sample will of necessity be self-selected or purposively sampled because of the need for telephone numbers. Responses collected through telephone interview should first be analysed separately from the main responses to eliminate any differences between the populations of postal replies and telephone replies. Only with the evidence that the two groups are indeed statistically similar should the two data sets be combined.

Prospective data collection

Retrospective data collection is unreliable because of the selective nature of memory. Ideally, prospective data collection should be used wherever possible, with observational validation of compliance. Data collection can be by tally counts, record or diary cards. Innovative methods such as taped self-report, or direct computer entry, possibly using a palm-top computer, should be considered. The easier the system is for the participant to integrate within their normal routine, the more complete and accurate will be the data collection. When designing data collection forms, similar principles should be followed to those described for designing questionnaire forms; questions must be clear and forms easy to follow. Forms should always be piloted before large-scale data collection exercises are started.

Experimental research

In the context of health services research, experimental research or empirical research method is normally used to demonstrate a causal effect between the introduction of a new treatment or management, and a defined outcome. Experimental research should be rigorously designed, with adequate controls, so that associations of intervention and outcome can be unequivocally stated. The two main methodological types are referred to as 'randomised controlled trials', in which eligible participants are allocated randomly to either the intervention or control group, and the two are compared to assess the effect of the new service offered, and 'before and after' studies, in which the same group is compared before and after the implementation of the new service. This latter method is weak because of the unknown effect of external factors. This can be partially overcome by the use of internal controls, for example by evaluating the outcome of a similar but distinct variable over the same time period.

Field research

Case study method Case study method is based primarily on observation and existing documentation. It is often used to follow novel developments and is very dependent on observation; non-participant and participant methods can be used. Objectivity and accuracy of data collection can be enhanced by use of validated instruments such as matrices of interactions (Bales, 1950) and taping of procedures (audio or video), as well as follow-up interviews with participants, and triangulation with formal documentation such as minutes. There are additional conflicting problems of confidentiality and ethics, due to the need to eliminate the 'Hawthorne' effect, which are difficult to resolve (Nisbet and Watt, 1980).

Interviews Interviews can be used as a means of administering a very structured questionnaire face to face, thus increasing individual response rate, ensuring that, wherever possible, all questions are answered, and allowing exploration of open questions. This has already been described. However, the full qualitative potential of the method is realised when the interviews are semi-structured or even completely unstructured. They are a useful research tool that can complement quantitative surveys, either at the beginning as content setting or at the end to add in-depth information to help explain other identified phenomena. This combination of techniques has been described by Moser and Kalton (1993) as providing a more powerful research strategy than reliance on any one method used alone. Standard methodology should always be followed (Powney and Watts, 1987; Moser and Kalton, 1993) when conducting interviews.

Open interviews can be alternatively described as qualitative, in-depth, semi-structured or focused. Such unstructured interviews fall along a scale of increasing formality (Moser and Kalton, 1993) ranging from the completely non-directive, when the interview is mainly guided by the interviewee, to the guided or focused interview. In the latter, although there is no set questionnaire, and most of the questions are open ones, the interviewee would be guided around predetermined topics. All individual interviewees should be provided with the same introductory information on the topic, but should then be free to develop various perspectives more or less dependent upon their own interests and to raise related topics not necessarily already identified as pertinent by the interviewer. Such interviews elicit both attitudes and factual information, and allow the respondents to cover various areas to differing extents. These interviews could also therefore be categorised as informant interviews (Powney and Watts, 1987).

The advantages of this type of information gathering, under these circumstances, are self-evident. There is a high response and it allows areas of interest to be developed and probed on an ad hoc basis. There are also disadvantages, the most important probably being dependence on the interviewer skills, interviewer bias, and interviewer variability. The interviewer–interviewee interaction, which may be one of rapport or the converse, could result in further bias, and in this latter respect the primary contact between the interviewer and interviewee has a major effect.

Analysis of open interviews is very different from the rigor of statistical methods used in quantitative work. It is essential to ensure that sufficient detail is retained to prevent the advantage of this methodology from being lost. This is well illustrated in Chapters 8 and 9.

Recording of interviews   Interviews are recorded using one of two main methods, either field note taking or tape recording with subsequent typed transcripts being used for analysis. The former has the disadvantage of intruding upon the interviewee's flow of thought, and the interviewer's concentration. Additionally, only a fraction of the total data can be recorded, although an advantage of this could be that these may be the key facts. Disadvantages are that accounts are biased by the interviewer's own 'mental set' at the time, and some facts may even consciously or subconsciously be ignored. In addition, the luxury of retrospective reflection of content is denied. Tape recording is complete and less intrusive, but results in resource implications for typing transcripts and lengthy documents for analysis.

There is a potential for bias in the interviews due to a variety of factors which may affect the way the interviewer directs, records and interprets the data. For example, these might include the perceptions and expectations of the interviewer as a result of both his/her own inherent opinions, and those formed from previous experimental work, previous interviews and previous knowledge of the current interviewee. This could lead to both an unconscious over-direction of the interview and a bias in the reporting of answers. In this respect the use of tape recording and verbatim transcription prior to analysis minimise these problems. Preconceptions on the part of the interviewer with respect to the respondent, as well as developing issues during the interview, might still have influenced the ordering of the issues, the emphasis and probing of different issues and even 'backing off' from points which appeared to be becoming controversial. Undue confrontation is considered to be detrimental to the remainder of the interview and therefore, in the wider context, better avoided.

Confidentiality in interviews   Wherever possible the interviewees should be contacted beforehand and given background information on the purpose of the interview, why they have been chosen and the likely time the interview will take. At the time of the interview the ground rules, including recording method and anonymity, and topics to be discussed, should be clearly explained and agreed. Respect for confidentiality regarding personal comments, or those subsequently withdrawn must be explicit. Wherever possible transcripts should be returned to the interviewee for approval. In studies where the interviewee is a public figure, the potential threat of exposure of ignorance, prejudice, apathy or intolerance has to be acknowledged. In general, no comments should be attributable to a named individual in the final distillation of the opinions.

Focus groups Focus groups are a form of group interview that is becoming increasingly widespread in its use (Pharmacy Practice Research Resource Centre, 1996; Kitzinger 1994; Barbour, 1995). Once again, they are a market research tool which has recently gained recognition in health services research and in other contexts. For example, there have recently been much publicised focus groups conducted in the UK by the Labour Party to identify the 'People's Agenda'. The benefit of focus groups is that they allow participants to say what they think, without the constraints of a structured schedule. The group facilitator has responsibility for setting the scene, with perhaps four sub-themes for the group to address, and he/she should try to ensure that all participants contribute to these. In a focus group new ideas will be generated because of interaction between the participants and this is a strength. It is important that participants are carefully selected to gain a range of opinions, and the exact method to achieve this will depend on the topic. Principles of recording and confidentiality are the same as for interviews.

Health economic aspects

One of the reasons pharmacy practice research was much criticised in the early report by Mays was because it appeared to be very focused on proving what pharmacists could do with respect to delivering new services. It was pointed out that what the research should really be showing was how well pharmacy could deliver a service compared with another model of delivery; for example, were pharmacists or practice nurses better at managing symptoms of minor ailments? It was also not necessarily just a case of demonstrating that pharmacists could deliver a specific service better than another profession, but also of considering whether or not it was cost effective to provide the service in this way.

Thus the net costs and benefits of the intervention had to be measured. These issues are dealt with in more detail in Chapter 4.

Data handling, storage and analysis

For small studies, data storage and analysis can be carried out using, pen, paper and calculator! The seminal work by Richard Doll linking lung cancer and smoking was done in this way. However, increasingly user-friendly computer software, access to personal computers, and spreadsheet, database and statistical packages all make data storage and manipulation quicker, more accurate and versatile. The simplest software, using EPI-info 5.0 (Dean *et al.*, 1990) is supported by the World Health Organization and is in the public domain; that means that any one can copy the program for their own use. Although now superseded by other programs, the basic statistical functions are all available and, for the first-time researcher with limited funds, it is an excellent tool. Beyond EPI-info there are many standard programs, the most widespread in use in pharmacy practice research currently being the Microsoft Office (Microsoft, 1992) suite of programs, which includes the database Access, and SPSS-PC (Norusis, 1993), a statistical package.

Simple descriptive statistics, such as frequencies, means, medians and modes, may often be all that is required. It is often interesting to look at associations between different variables, and for this, parametric tests such as analysis of variance, and non-parametric tests such as the chi-square, are often used. The Wilcoxon paired t-test, used to demonstrate differences between two samples, is another commonly applied procedure.

Ethical approval

Traditionally, the need to seek ethical approval for studies in which the subjects were submitted to new treatments and invasive tests was self-evident. Such approval is normally given by a local ethical committee which includes multidisciplinary and lay representatives. More recently, the administration of a postal questionnaire or interview is seen to be intrusive on a person's privacy and nearly all studies involving patients in any way now require ethical approval. This approval will consider the way in which patients are identified, the information they receive and the mechanism for obtaining informed consent, and the content of any questionnaire or interview schedule. Because ethical committees are normally geographically located, the need to seek multiple approvals when conducting a national study has presented a formidable workload at the start of a study. For this reason, and to reduce workload on individual ethical committees, new Multicentre Research Ethics Committees (MRECs) have been created for Scotland. Once they have approved a study, all that is needed is for local committees to decide whether or not to allow it to take place in their area; they do not re-assess it per se. In theory this is a good idea, but it is still in its infancy and, to date, there are anecdotal reports of local committees still wishing to make changes to protocols to meet their individual local requirements.

Feedback to participants

Ideally, results should be fed back to the participants wherever possible. This may be more as a matter of courtesy than for gain for the researcher or methodological need. It is generally hoped that the results will be of interest to the participants and stimulate their further support. However, feedback can also provide additional data and research opportunity.

   In large national surveys resources may not always allow feedback to individual participants and feedback/dissemination may be best achieved by timely publication of the results in both academic and professional journals. To date the choice of journal has been mostly limited to either a pharmacy journal (*Pharmaceutical Journal, International Journal of Pharmacy Practice, Journal of Social and Administrative Pharmacy*), or a medical journal, such as the *British Medical Journal* or the *British Journal of General Practice*. Issues of relevance and quality, as well as space and topicality, have highlighted the need for a wider range of multidisciplinary journals and a few such journals are now being published (e.g. *Quality in Health Care*).

Conclusion

Evidence is essential to inform the development of professional practice and make recommendations for changes in models of healthcare delivery. However, it is important that the evidence is considered critically, and the weight placed on it coloured by the robustness of the methods used. It is also important to be aware of the developing discipline of health services research, and thereby practice research, and to be aware that studies conducted to the best standards even five years ago will not necessarily pass the required quality criteria today. This is because our understanding of the necessary techniques has developed, and also because those funding health services research are more informed on the necessary processes and their resource implications. Thus, we can design studies with a reduced need to continually minimise costs at the expense of the design.

Some of the studies reported in these chapters were conducted in the early days of pharmacy practice research and would not necessarily be done in the same way today. These points are acknowledged where appropriate. However, it is still of value to record these studies in this volume because, at the time, they were pushing forward the methodology for practice research, raising awareness of the science and, most importantly, informing the future of our profession, with the best data then available.

References

Anonymous (1992a). Royal College of GPs accepts pharmacy report with reservations. *Pharm J* 249: 305.

Anonymous (1992b). Profession welcomes working party report. *Pharm J* 248: 314.

Anonymous (1992c). No pipe dream. *Pharm J* 248: 305.

Anonymous (1998). Fifty years of randomised controlled trials. *BMJ* 317.

Bales R F (1950). *Interaction process analysis: a method for the study of small groups*. Cambridge, Mass: Addison-Wesley.

Barber N, Smith F, Anderson S (1994). Improving quality of health care: the role of pharmacists. *Quality in Health Care* 3: 153–58.

Barbour R S (1995). Using focus groups in general practice research. *Fam Pract* 12: 328–34.

Bero L A, Mays N B, Bond C M, *et al.* (1997). Expanding pharmacists' roles and health services utilisation, costs and patient outcomes. *Cochrane Database of Reviews*.

Bond C M (1999). Pharmacy and primary healthcare. In: Sims J, ed. *Primary Health Care Sciences*, London: Whurr.

Cotter S M, Barber N D, McKee M (1994). Professionalisation of hospital pharmacy: the role of clinical pharmacy. *J Soc Admin Pharm* 11(2): 57–66.

Dean A G, Dean J A, Burton A H, *et al.* (1990). *Epi Info Version 5: A Word Processing, Database and Statistics System for Epidemiology on Microcomputers*. USD Incorporated, 2075A West Park Place, Stone Mountain, Georgia.

Department of Health (1992). *Pharmaceutical care: the future for community pharmacy*. London: Royal Pharmaceutical Society of Great Britain.

Department of Health (1997). *The New NHS: modern and dependable*. Cm 3807 London: HMSO.

Dickersin K, Manheimer E (1998). The Cochrane Collaboration: evaluation of health care and services using systematic reviews of the results of randomised controlled trials. *Clin Obstet Gynecol* 41(2): 315–331.

Eaton G, Webb B (1979). Boundary encroachment: pharmacists in the clinical setting. *Sociol Health Illness* 1(1): 69–89.

Green J, Britten N (1998). Qualitative research and evidence based medicine. *BMJ* 316: 1230–32.

Kitzinger J (1994). The methodology of focus groups: the importance of interaction between research participants. *Sociol Health Illness* 16: 103–21.

Mays (1994). *Health services research in pharmacy: a critical personal review*. London: King's Fund.

Medical Research Council (1993). *The Medical Research Council Scientific Strategy*. London: Medical Research Council.

Merrison A W (1979). *Royal Commission on the National Health Service*. Cmnd 7615. London: HMSO.

Microsoft (1992). *Access Relational Database Management System for Windows user's guide*. Richmond, VA: Microsoft Corporation.

Moser C A, Kalton G (1993). *Survey methods in social investigation*. Aldershot: Dartmouth Publishing Company Ltd.

Nisbet J, Watt J (1982). *Case Study: Rediguide 26. Guides in Educational Research*. Nottingham: Nottingham University.

Norusis M (1993). *SPSS for Windows Base System User's Guide Release 6.0*. Chicago, IL: SPSS Inc.

Oppenheim A N (1993). *Questionnaire design, interviewing and attitude measurement*. London: Pinter Publishers Ltd.

Pharmacy Practice Research Conference Proceedings (1991). *Action in practice research*. London: Department of Health and Royal Pharmaceutical Society of Great Britain.

Pharmacy Practice Research Resource Centre (1992). Designing and administering questionnaires. *Pharmacy Practice Research Resource Centre Bulletin* 1(1): 3. Manchester: Pharmacy Practice Research Resource Centre.

Pharmacy Practice Research Resource Centre (1996). Spotlight on focus groups. *Pharmacy Practice Research Resource Centre Bulletin* 5.3. Manchester: Pharmacy Practice Research Resource Centre.

Pharmacy Practice Research Resource Centre (1997). *The pharmacy practice research enterprise scheme: a resource document*. Manchester: Pharmacy Practice Research Resource Centre.

Pharmacy Practice Research Task Force (1997). *A new age for pharmacy practice research: promoting evidence-based practice in pharmacy*. London: Royal Pharmaceutical Society of Great Britain.

Powney J, Watts M (1987). *Interviewing in educational research*. London: Routledge.

Royal Pharmaceutical Society of Great Britain (1997a). A new age for pharmacy practice research. Promoting evidence based practice in pharmacy. *Report of the pharmacy practice R and D task force*. London: Royal Pharmaceutical Society of Great Britain.

Royal Pharmaceutical Society of Great Britain (1997b). Investing in evidence based practice in pharmacy. *A summary of the report produced by the pharmacy practice R and D task force*. London: Royal Pharmaceutical Society of Great Britain.

Scottish Health Service Management Executive (1997). *Primary care: agenda for action*. Edinburgh: Scottish Office Department of Health.

Secretary of State for Scotland (1997). *Designed to care: renewing the National Health Service in Scotland*. CM 3811. Edinburgh: Scottish Office Department of Health.

Secretary of State for Wales (1998). *NHS Wales – putting patients first*. CM 3841. London: The Stationery Office.

Smith M C, Knapp D A (1972). *Pharmacy, drugs, and medical care*. Baltimore: Williams and Wilkins.

Taylor R J (1992). *A novel method for identifying questionnaire returns whilst retaining anonymity*. Personal communication.

Taylor R J, Alexander D A, Fordyce I D (1986). A survey of paramenstrual complaints by covert and by overt methods. *J R Coll Gen Pract* 36: 496–99.

Trease G E (1965). In Poynter F N L, ed. *The evolution of pharmacy in Britain*. London: Pitman Medical Publishing.

2

Advice-giving in community pharmacy

Felicity Smith

Introduction

Health services are continually evolving in response to new healthcare priorities, population needs and demands. Technological development and demographic and societal change require the health service and individual professional groups to reappraise their activities to ensure the continued provision of effective and appropriate services.

Pharmacy is no exception. Although advice-giving has remained a prominent feature of pharmacists' roles throughout a long history, their advice-giving activities must continually evolve in response to changes in health service structures and provision, expectations and wishes of clients, outlooks of fellow health professionals and Government health policy agendas and priorities.

The Royal Pharmaceutical Society of Great Britain (RPSGB) launched the Pharmacy in the New Age (PIANA) initiative to encourage debate within the profession regarding the future of pharmacy services and promote innovation appropriate to the changing demands, expectations and outlooks regarding future healthcare provision (RPSGB, 1996a; RPSGB, 1996b). Advice-giving is central to all five areas identified in this strategy (RPSGB, 1997a): the management of prescribed medicines, the management of long-term conditions, the management of common ailments, the promotion and support of healthy lifestyles and advice and support for other healthcare professionals. The strategy emphasises the important role of individual pharmacists in actively identifying new directions for pharmacy services (RPSGB, 1998). The Royal Pharmaceutical Society (1997b) is also promoting the concept of concordance to describe and encourage a framework in which there is partnership between patients and professionals in decisions about healthcare and drug therapy. A change in approach from compliance to concordance would also be expected to have implications for advice-giving in pharmacies.

Service development must be in accordance with changing government policies and priorities for the future of healthcare. In their emphasis on health promotion (to address the high levels of morbidity and mortality from diseases for which 'lifestyle' risk factors are well known) the Government is seeking to encourage people to take more responsibility for their own health (Secretary of State for Health, 1999). The potential role of pharmacy in health promotion has been well recognised by the profession. Reclassification of drugs from prescription-only to non-prescription may provide opportunities for individuals to manage their own common ailments without recourse to medical services. This also presents new opportunities for pharmacists, and demands by clients, regarding advice-giving in the pharmacy.

Promoting high quality healthcare and uniformity of standards across Britain is a priority of Government policy. A National Institute for Clinical Excellence (NICE) has been established to set national standards as part of the Government's strategy to ensure high quality services throughout the health service (Government White Paper, 1998; Harman, 1999). It is intended that local standards will be developed alongside these national guidelines. Clinical governance, which has been defined as 'a framework through which NHS organisations are accountable for continuously improving the quality of their services and safeguarding high standards of care by creating an environment in which excellence in clinical care can flourish' (Government White Paper, 1998) has become an important focus for the development of procedures to ensure that Government objectives are met. The professional isolation of community pharmacists has been highlighted many times as a hindrance to the development of co-ordinated services. However, in line with other sectors of healthcare, measures to ensure high quality and more uniform standards should be adopted within pharmacy services.

It is proposed that guidelines produced by NICE will be evidence-based, drawing on systematic reviews of research. The increasing emphasis on evidence-based practice must also apply to pharmacy. Advice-giving should be both based on the best available evidence and appropriate to the client's needs. Clinical studies have assumed an important role in providing information for evidence-based practice. However, the Government's strategy of quality assurance includes an annual survey of patient and user experiences of the health service (Department of Health, 1998). To achieve optimal outcomes from the perspectives of patients, an evidence-base is required on those features of healthcare (including advice-giving) that are valued by patients.

As pharmacy advisory services evolve and innovations are implemented, appropriate evaluation is important to ensure the provision of relevant and high quality healthcare.

Methodological problems and issues

Components of advice-giving

Evidence-based medicine, which has been defined as 'the conscientious, explicit and judicious use of current best evidence in making decisions about the care of individual patients' (Sackett *et al.*, 1996) is now viewed as a means of ensuring the most effective healthcare. Evidence-based practice requires data which provide information on alternative approaches to care and/or treatment options. In the case of advice-giving, such evidence would assist practitioners in ensuring their advice-giving practices are in accordance with principles known to result in optimal outcomes.

In examining advice-giving, researchers have distinguished separate clinical and communicative aspects. Studies have focused on describing and evaluating both the content of the advice and the processes of communication.

In terms of the content of advice, clinical studies can evaluate alternative treatment options on the basis of clinical outcomes and provide evidence on the relative effectiveness of different therapies or courses of action. For many symptoms and conditions, there will also be relevant information on health promotion and disease prevention activities which would be expected to lead to improved health outcomes. The content of advice can be devised accordingly.

However, clinical input is just one factor on which advice-giving should be assessed. The processes of advice-giving are also an important determinant of the quality of advice. The advantages and disadvantages of different styles of questioning, and the levels of involvement of the professional and client in decision-making is believed to affect outcomes in terms of patient satisfaction and adherence (RPSGB, 1997b). Increasingly, emphasis is placed on involving patients in decisions about their healthcare. Guadagnoli and Ward (1998), in their review of patient participation in decision making, did not feel that the benefits had been demonstrated in research. However, they believed that the evidence showed that patients generally wished to be more involved and that, in doing so, practitioners may well be improving the effectiveness of care in terms of serving the patient's goals.

For effective health promotion, in particular, it is generally acknowledged that advice must be relevant to people's lives, outlooks and priorities. Thus, in the process of advising, receptiveness and responsiveness to the client's perspectives will be of paramount importance.

Each interaction between a client and health professional is unique. The issues raised in the consultation, the information provided and the communicative processes should be based on evidence of association with optimal health outcomes. These features should also be pertinent to the particular needs and expectations of each client. Acknowledgement of responsibility for health outcomes is a central feature of pharmaceutical care. This requires a professional service which identifies and addresses these unique needs of individual clients.

Assessing outcomes of advice-giving

Outcomes attributable to advice-giving may be multifactorial. Just as studies have revealed differences between the public and health professionals in their views regarding healthcare priorities (Bowling, 1993), professionals and the public will have their own thoughts on the goals of advice-giving. Health professionals may be most concerned with clinical outcomes, health policy-makers may be keen that advice-giving on common ailments becomes an accepted alternative to consultation with medical practitioners. Health economists may focus on the purchase of non-prescription medicines leading to a reduction in prescription costs (see Chapter 4). The greatest concerns to clients may be the waiting time for the advice and the privacy afforded, rather than the content of the advice itself. Direct or indirect costs to patients of the actions and their consequences may also be an important issue in their evaluation.

Thus, for any single interaction, the pharmacist and the client will have their own views regarding the goals and anticipated outcomes. These may include the alleviation of symptoms, the promotion of a behavioural change, reassurance, to obtain or provide specific items of information, to improve adherence to a course of action, or to provide information to enable the client to make their own decisions.

As summarised in Chapter 1, randomised controlled trials are believed to provide the strongest evidence of efficacy of healthcare interventions. The strength of these studies lies in the experimental design which enables the assessment of alternative treatment options between groups similar in all respects save the alternative treatment options. Thus, differences in outcomes between the groups can be assumed to be directly attributable to the treatment option.

Although randomised controlled trials are common in evaluating the relative clinical efficacy of different treatment options, for many of the alternative courses of action or drug therapies for the management of common symptoms, evidence is limited.

Few researchers have attempted experimental studies to evaluate the outcomes of advice-giving in community pharmacy. The application of randomised controlled trials to advice-giving in community settings presents both practical and ethical difficulties for researchers. For example, imposing standardised advice-giving procedures may be seen by both health professionals and clients as potentially compromising the quality of professional services, or limiting opportunities for incorporating the client's preferences and concerns in decisions regarding the advice-giving process.

Measurement of specific outcomes can also present methodological difficulties. In studies which involve following up clients to establish the extent to which advice was followed or the symptoms were alleviated, outcomes may be difficult to quantify and the extent to which they are attributable to the antecedent advice may also be difficult to verify. In many instances, valid and reliable tools for the measurement of relevant outcomes may not be available.

In assessing interventions, many researchers would want to show an impact on the health status of the client: to demonstrate an improvement in the health-related quality of life of the individual rather than focusing on a clinical measure (which may or may not be a reliable reflection of improved health status and its consequences). Many measures have now been developed for this purpose and they are widely employed. They necessarily include a subjective component in that they are related to an individual's own feelings rather than being determined by external factors which can be 'objectively' measured. These measures have not been designed for the assessment of the impact of advice-giving in pharmacies. Suitable measures would be those sensitive to specific and anticipated outcomes relevant to health problems presented in pharmacy settings.

Donabedian has stressed the importance of assessing satisfaction with healthcare as it provides an indication of the extent to which clients' expectations and wishes are achieved (Donabedian, 1980; Donabedian 1992). Client satisfaction is increasingly used as an indicator of quality in health services, despite problems in its measurement. An annual survey of patient and user experiences of the NHS forms part of the Government's strategy of quality assurance in health services (Government White Paper, 1998). Patient satisfaction is structurally complex. It comprises many components some more important to the overall attribute, and particular clients, than others. Furthermore, reported satisfaction is known to change over time (Carr-Hill, 1992). Demonstrating that a series of questions is a reliable and valid measure of an individual's beliefs and experiences is problematic.

Structure, process and outcome

A framework for the assessment of healthcare interventions has been presented by Donabedian based on the separate consideration of the structures of services, processes in their delivery and the outcomes of care (Donabedian, 1980). The difficulties of measuring outcomes has led researchers to evaluate services (including advisory services) in terms of the structure and process components, assuming a relationship between these components and outcomes.

Donabedian does not view structure (appropriate resources and system design) as a measure of quality of care, but he argues that the structural characteristics of the healthcare setting will influence the process of care and hence its quality; he also views appropriate structures as the most important means of protecting and promoting good quality care. Thus, without appropriate structures and processes based on the best available evidence, optimal outcomes (attributable to the intervention) would be unlikely to result.

Randomised controlled trials are not appropriate for investigating the impact of structural factors (e.g. features of buildings, environment, organisation and staff) many of which are fixed. Bowling (1997) suggests that the most suitable approach is a descriptive survey in which the data are collected within an experimental design to compare these factors in relation to outcome.

Many assessments of advice-giving have focused on the processes of the interaction; the processes being seen as a prerequisite and/or a proxy for outcomes. Just as suitable structural features may be important determinants for optimal outcomes, the processes in the delivery of care must also be appropriate. A study of the relationship between structure (services and management) and processes (conduct of doctor–patient consultations) in a general medical practice setting concluded that structure and process may contribute to patient outcomes independently of each other (Ram et al., 1998).

In developing and assessing healthcare, the Government is keen to ensure that services (structures and processes) are responsive to the priorities and needs of patients. Structural components (e.g. accessibility and privacy) and processes of advice-giving (style and conduct of the consultation) are known to be important issues to clients in determining whether or not the client's goals are achieved (Smith and Salkind 1988; Smith, 1990; Hedvall and Paltschik, 1991; Williamson *et al.*, 1992; Krska *et al.* 1995; Hassell *et al.*, 1998). Thus, as well as a means to an end, the processes of care themselves may be an important component of the desired outcome.

Research studies

Obtaining and validating data

Methods of data-collection to study advice-giving in community pharmacy have included self-completion surveys, diaries and direct observation by a researcher. All methods have their own strengths and weaknesses in terms of the feasibility of data collection and the reliability and validity of the information. Ortiz *et al.* (1989) compared the data on advice-giving collected by different methods and found that, in general, self-completion questionnaires over-estimated the frequency and duration of episodes, whilst diaries tended to over-estimate duration but under-estimate the frequency; direct observation was believed to have little impact on activities.

Many studies of advice-giving have involved observation by researchers who remain in the pharmacy for set periods. The presence of the observer however discreet, may influence the behaviours of the individuals being observed resulting in data of questionable validity (although Ortiz *et al.* (1989) found only a minimal impact). Observers have attempted to minimise this effect by e.g., wearing non-uniform clothes or positioning themselves as unobtrusively as possible whilst still able to collect all the relevant data (Taylor and Suveges, 1992; Stevenson and Taylor, 1995). Researchers have also devised methods to assess the extent of bias caused by the research process; for instance, by collecting data by two different methods and comparing the results (Smith and Salkind, 1990) or by involving counter staff in collecting additional data for a specified period, the pharmacist not being informed of the timing of this period (Aslanpour and Smith, 1997). Some researchers have employed covert methods to collect data, in particular, the deployment of 'pseudo-patients' who present in pharmacies claiming to be experiencing particular symptoms and recording certain details of the response of the pharmacy staff (Consumers' Association 1985; Consumers' Association 1991; Anderson and Alexander, 1992).

Direct observation by a researcher located in the pharmacy for the duration of the data collection is necessary to collect comprehensive data. Manual transcription at the time of the consultation presents inevitable problems in terms of obtaining a detailed record of a verbal exchange due to inaudibility of some consultations and intrusiveness of the researcher who has to be placed in close proximity to the pharmacist and client. To overcome these problems, a number of investigators have audio-taped consultations (Smith *et al.*, 1990; Smith 1992; Wilson *et al.*, 1992; Evans and John, 1997; Blom *et al.*, 1998; Pilnick, 1998). The use of radio-microphone apparatus worn by the pharmacist enables a full record of interactions wherever they occur in the pharmacy but restricts the data collection to consultations involving the person wearing the microphone. The data obtained include only the verbal content of the interaction and do not allow analysis relating to environmental or contextual factors which may be important to the processes and outcomes of the interaction. Tape-recordings have been used to provide data for both quantitative and qualitative analysis of pharmacist–client interactions.

Video-taping of consultations has also been undertaken in community pharmacy. This approach is less common possibly because of the logistical and ethical issues it presents. However, it has the advantage over other methods in that data collected enable a consideration of both verbal and non-verbal communication (Hargie *et al.*, 1993).

To ensure the collection of data representative of advice-giving in pharmacy as a whole, the data collection must be planned to include: sufficient numbers of pharmacies, appropriate sampling procedures, timing and duration of data collection periods to include different times of day, week and possibly year. This can be difficult to achieve in observation studies which are relatively costly in terms of researcher time and resources.

Study design

Studies to investigate and evaluate advice-giving in community pharmacies have mostly been descriptive studies: characterising advice-giving and exploring associated factors. Much of this research has incorporated the collection of data on structural factors to assess their relationship with aspects of the advisory role; these have included comparing different types of pharmacy (e.g., independent, small and large multiple), location of the pharmacy (urban, rural) characteristics of the pharmacist (e.g., age, sex, occupational status), the clientele (predominantly regular or casual), or prescription throughput. Some studies have aimed to identify factors associated with the number of requests for advice and the extent of advice-giving. Exploration of associations reveals complex relationships between variables. Many studies are also localised and the findings are not necessarily transferable to other areas. Structural features of pharmacy services are commonly cited as a restraint on advice-giving activities and a study into barriers to the extension of the advisory activities of community pharmacists following legislative changes found structural features to be a barrier to service development (Barnes *et al.*, 1996). Raisch (1993) in a descriptive study carried out in New Mexico, USA found a relationship between counselling and prescription payment systems, although some of the variables were confounded in that pharmacies with higher numbers of capitation patients (who received less advice) were those with high workloads. Capitation patients were those who were enrolled at a particular pharmacy, and for whom the pharmacy was reimbursed by a specified amount regardless of the level of use of prescription services.

In assessing the quality of advice, many researchers have focused on process variables (i.e., gathering data on the advice provided and its delivery) as proxies for outcomes. Thus, in assessing the quality of advice researchers have assessed the content of advice and looked for features in the communication which would be expected to result in, or be a prerequisite for, positive outcomes. Studies by the Consumers' Association and a number of other researchers (Consumers' Association 1985; Consumers' Association 1991; Anderson and Alexander, 1992; Krska *et al.*, 1994) have involved pseudo-patients and focused on the content, i.e. whether or not pharmacy staff asked particular questions and provided specific items of advice (believed by a panel of experts to be important). Other researchers have employed methodologies that have enabled the investigation of characteristics of the communication between pharmacists and clients, such as assessments of the style of questioning, degree of explanation, attention to concerns and questions of clients, input by the pharmacist and the client (Smith *et al.*, 1990; Smith, 1992; Morrow *et al.*, 1993; Evans and John, 1995; Pilnick 1998). Aspects such as the privacy afforded by the consultation area have also been highlighted. Studies involving 'pseudo-patients' allow an assessment only in accordance with the pre-set criteria determined by the researchers. They do not enable an assessment of communication skills in the context of the varying conditions and circumstances in which they may arise.

A study by Morrow and Hargie (1987) employed a qualitative technique to characterise factors which are important to the interpersonal process. Critical incident methodology enabled the identification of difficult cases from which a wide range of problems and issues were described.

Deriving criteria of assessment

The evaluation of advice-giving requires agreement regarding the features against which advice-giving should be assessed. 'Expert panels' or consensus methods such as the Delphi method or the nominal group technique (Hunter and Jones, 1995; Cantrill *et al.*, 1996) have been employed for this purpose. These techniques have been used to establish priorities from the perspective of health professionals regarding advice-giving in the pharmacy (Smith *et al.*, 1990). Other approaches have been applied to investigate the views of clients regarding important features of consultations and advice-giving in pharmacy (Smith and Salkind, 1988; Smith, 1990; Hedvall and Paltschik, 1991; Williamson *et al.*, 1992; Krska *et al.*, 1995; Hassell *et al.*, 1998).

In the study by Hargie *et al.* (1993), video-consultations between pharmacists and their clients provided a basis from which pharmacists distinguished issues on which they believed consultations should be assessed. This resulted in a list of skills and subskills, but also enabled the identification of a range of situation-specific issues.

Individual consultations or interactions can then be assessed regarding the extent to which each of these features are displayed. Visual analogue or Likert scales are commonly employed in the rating of interventions and possible outcomes. Reliability between the ratings of different assessors is an issue addressed by many researchers. Because the assessment of any interaction is recognised as involving a subjective component, researchers wish to demonstrate that the scores assigned by different raters are reflective of differences between the interactions and not merely a result of varying perceptions and value judgements of the assessors. To improve reliability, rating scales should include clear definitions of the criteria against which the interactions are to be assessed and researchers should check for uniform interpretation of these by different assessors.

Despite these precautions, it is to be expected that assessors would vary to some extent in their ratings, and assign different scores. There may also be variation between scores assigned on repeated occasions by the same individuals or as a result of other external factors. Generalisability theory can be used to quantify and address this variation, or subjectivity, in the evaluation of healthcare.

Generalisability theory enables the identification of sources of error in assessments and the design of a study to take account of it. For example, variation in assessments of interactions may be due to differences of opinion of those conducting the assessment, poor reliability of scales used, or the perspectives of different professional groups. The first stage of generalisability theory comprises a factorial experiment in which the error attributable to these multiple sources can be estimated in terms of several variance components (Cronbach *et al.*, 1963). Once identified and quantified, further assessments can be designed to reduce the unwanted variation (Cronbach *et al.*, 1972). The application of this method enables the researcher to select operational conditions for the assessment of advice-giving which controls for subjectivity in the assessment, thus providing results of known generalisability. Generalisability theory has been applied to many issues in different settings including pharmacy studies (Smith *et al.*, 1990; Smith *et al.*, 1995; Dean and Barber, 1999). For the assessment of advice-giving in pharmacies, operational conditions (numbers of assessors and judgements) can be selected so that a generalisability coefficient of approximately 0.8 would be achieved on each criterion (Smith *et al.*, 1990).

Outcomes

Some researchers have attempted to assess specific outcomes of advice-giving in community pharmacy. In these studies, data relating to the consultation have been collected by observation and/or audio-tape and the clients followed-up by questionnaire or interview to establish subsequent actions and outcomes. These include assessments of the extent to which clients could recall information given (Wilson *et al.*, 1992), the extent to which advice was reported to have been followed (Evans *et al.*, 1997) and whether or not advice to see a general practitioner resulted in a consultation (Blenkinsopp *et al.*, 1991). The feasibility of diaries, maintained by clients, for recording outcomes following the purchase of non-prescription medicines has also been explored (Cantrill *et al.*, 1995).

The majority of referrals made by community pharmacists when advising on symptoms are made to general medical practitioners. The referral practices of pharmacists in terms of the nature and duration of symptoms referred has been assessed from the perspective of general practitioners (Smith, 1996).

Few researchers have undertaken experimental studies to evaluate aspects of advice-giving. A before-and-after study was conducted to assess the effect of a shop-front pharmacist on non-prescription medicine consultations. Data collected prior to, and following, the placement of a pharmacist at the front of the shop documented an increase in consultations between the study periods (Stevenson and Taylor, 1995). A similar study design was used to evaluate the impact of a training workshop on the process of advice-giving by pharmacists (Berado *et al.*, 1989).

A randomised-controlled trial was conducted by Rantucci and Segal (1985) to assess outcome and effectiveness of patient counselling in community pharmacy. Clients purchasing non-prescription medicines were assigned randomly to either a control or study group which determined whether or not they received counselling. Subsequent telephone interviews were then conducted to assess the outcome of the counselling with respect to the client's knowledge of the medication and the appropriateness of its use.

The future

The Government has emphasised the importance of ensuring quality through the provision of evidence-based care. This included incorporating evidence into, and disseminating correspondingly high standards through, national and local guidelines.

Many researchers have undertaken descriptive studies into aspects of advice-giving in community pharmacy, and a number of attempts have been made to assess the quality of advice in terms of structures of services, and processes and outcomes of advice-giving. These studies have employed different approaches to overcome some of the methodological problems. Few studies of advice-giving have demonstrated the relative effectiveness of different approaches. Although structural features and processes of care may be seen as pre-requisites for optimal outcomes, the actual relationships between these aspects of care remain unclear.

Advice-giving must be evaluated in the context of a wide range of client, public, professional, health policy goals and outcomes. Sackett (1996) in his definition and discussion of evidence-based medicine identifies the importance of addressing the needs of individual clients in its application. Aspects of structure of services and processes of care may be important in themselves as well as a means to achieving a particular clinical outcome.

The direction of professional development suggests that advice-giving with medicines and on common ailments will remain a prominent and important feature of pharmacy services. Advice-giving is central to all the five areas identified in the RPSGB strategy for community pharmacy (RPSGB, 1997a). Changing perspectives in advice-giving will lead to new agendas and approaches in research; these may include the examination and differentiation of patterns and styles of communication, the evaluation of advice-giving in the wider the context of pharmacy settings and the development of measures for specific anticipated outcomes.

References

Anderson C W, Alexander A M (1992). Response to dysmenorrhoea: an assessment of knowledge and skills. *Pharm J* 249: R2.

Aslanpour Z, Smith F J (1997). Oral counselling on dispensed medication: a survey of its extent and associated factors in a random sample of community pharmacies. *Int J Pharm Pract* 5: 57–63.

Barnes J M, Riedlinger J E, McCloskey W W, *et al.* (1996). Barriers to compliance with OBRA'90 regulations in community pharmacies. *Ann Pharmacother* 30: 1101–05.

Berardo D H, Kimberlin C L, Barnett C W (1989). Observational research on patient activities of community pharmacists. *J Soc Admin Pharm* 6: 21–30.

Blenkinsopp A, Jepson M H, Drury M (1991). Using a notification card to improve communication between community pharmacists and general medical practitioners. *Br J Gen Pract* 41: 116–18.

Blom L, Jonkers R, Kok G, *et al.* (1998). Patient education in 20 Dutch pharmacies: analysis of audiotaped contacts. *Int J Pharm Pract* 6: 72–76.

Bowling A (1993). *What people say about prioritising health services*. London: King's Fund Centre.

Bowling A (1997). *Research Methods in Health*. Buckingham: Open University Press.

Cantrill J A, Sibbald B, Buetow S (1996). The Delphi and nominal group technique in health services research. *Int J Pharm Pract* 4: 67–74.

Cantrill J A, Vaezi L, Nicolson M, *et al.* (1995). A study to explore the feasibility of using a health diary to monitor therapeutic outcomes from over-the-counter medicines. *J Soc Admin Pharm* 12: 190–98.

Carr-Hill R A (1992). The measurement of patient satisfaction. *J Public Health Med* 14: 236–49.

Consumers' Association (1985). Advice across a chemist's counter. *Which?* August: 351–54.

Consumers' Association (1991). Pharmacists: how reliable are they? *Which? Way to Health* December: 191–94.

Cronbach L J, Rajaratnam N, Gleser G C (1963). Theory of generalisability: a liberalisation of reliability theory. *British Journal of Statistical Psychology* 16: 137–63.

Cronbach L J, Gleser G C, Harinda Nanda A N, *et al.* (1972). *The dependability of behavioural measurements: theory of generalisability for scores and profiles*. New York: Wiley.

Dean B S, Barber N D (1999). A validated, reliable method of scoring the severity of medication errors. *Am J Health Syst Pharm* 56: 57–62.

Department of Health (1998). *A first class service: quality in the new NHS*. London: Department of Health.

Donabedian A (1980). *Explorations in quality assessment and monitoring volume 1: The definition of quality and approaches to its assessment*. Michigan: Health Administration Press.

Donabedian A (1992). Quality assurance in healthcare: consumers' role. *Quality in Health Care* 1: 247–51.

Evans S W, John D N (1995). A preliminary investigation of the interactions between UK and US community pharmacists and their prescription clients. *Int J Pharm Pract* 3: 157–62.

Evans S W, John D N, Bloor M J, *et al.* (1997). Use of non-prescription advice offered to the public by community pharmacists. *Int J Pharm Pract* 5: 16–25.

Guadagnoli E, Ward P (1998). Patient participation in decision-making. *Soc Sci Med* 47: 329–39.

Hargie O D W, Morrow N, Woodman C (1993). *Looking into community pharmacy: identifying effective communication skills in pharmacist-patient consultations.* Belfast: The Queen's University of Belfast.

Harman R J (1999). The National Institute for Clinical Excellence. *Pharm J* 263: 869–76.

Hassell K, Noyce P, Rogers A, *et al.* (1998). Advice provided in British community pharmacies: what people want and what they get. *Journal of Health Services Research and Policy* 3: 219–25.

Hedvall M-B, Paltschik M (1991). Developing pharmacy services: customer driven interaction and counselling approach. *Service Industries Journal* 11: 36–46.

Hunter D, Jones J (1995). Consensus methods for medical and health services research. *BMJ* 311: 376–80.

Krska J, Greenwood R, Howitt E P (1994). Audit of advice provided in response to symptoms. *Pharm J* 252: 93–96.

Krska J, Kennedy E M, Milne S A, *et al.* (1995). Frequency of counselling on prescription medicines in community pharmacy. *Int J Pharm Pract* 3: 178–85.

Morrow N C, Hargie O D W (1987). An investigation of critical incidents in interpersonal communication in pharmacy practice. *J Soc Admin Pharm* 4: 112–20.

Morrow N C, Hargie O D W, Donnelly H, *et al.* (1993). 'Why do you ask?' A study of questioning behaviour in community pharmacy-client consultations. *Int J Pharm Pract* 2: 90–94.

Ortiz M, Walker W L, Thomas R (1989). Comparisons between methods of assessing patient counselling in Australian community pharmacies. *J Soc Admin Pharm* 6: 39–48.

Pilnick A (1998). 'Why didn't you just say that?' Dealing with issues of asymmetry, knowledge and competence in the pharmacist/client encounter. *Sociol Health Illness* 20: 29–51.

Raisch D W (1993). Patient counselling in community pharmacy and its relationship with prescription payment methods and practice settings. *Ann Pharmacother* 27: 1173–79.

Ram P, Grol R, van den Hombergh P, *et al.* (1998). Structure and process: the relationship between practice management and actual clinical performance in general practice. *Fam Pract* 15: 354–62.

Rantucci M J, Segal H J (1985). Over-the-counter medication: outcome and effectiveness of patient counselling. *J Soc Admin Pharm* 3: 81–91.

Royal Pharmaceutical Society of Great Britain (1996a). *Pharmacy in a new age: developing a strategy for the future. A discussion paper.* London: RPSGB.

Royal Pharmaceutical Society of Great Britain (1996b). *Pharmacy in a new age: the new horizon. A consultation on the future of the profession.* London: RPSGB.

Royal Pharmaceutical Society of Great Britain (1997a). *Pharmacy in a new age. Building the future: a strategy for a 21st century pharmaceutical service.* London: RPSGB.

Royal Pharmaceutical Society of Great Britain (1997b). *From compliance to concordance: achieving shared goals in medicine taking.* London: RPSGB.

Royal Pharmaceutical Society of Great Britain (1998). *Pharmacy in a new age. Over to you: helping pharmacists shape their professional future.* London: RPSGB.

Sackett D L, Rosenburg W M, Gray J A M, *et al.* (1996). Evidence-based medicine: what it is and what it is not. *BMJ* 312: 71–72.

Secretary of State for Health (1999). *Saving lives: our healthier nation.* CM 4386. London: HMSO.

Smith F J (1990). Factors important to clients when seeking the advice of a pharmacist. *Pharm J* 244: 692–93.

Smith F J (1992). Community pharmacists and health promotion: a study of consultations between pharmacists and clients. *Health Promotion International* 7: 249–55.

Smith F J (1996). Referral of clients by community pharmacists: views of general medical practitioners. *Int J Pharm Pract* 4: 30–35.

Smith F J, Salkind M R (1988). Counselling areas in community pharmacies: views of pharmacists and clients. *Pharm J* 241: R7.

Smith F J, Salkind M R (1990). Factors influencing the extent of the pharmacist's advisory role in Greater London. *Pharm J* 244: R4–R7.

Smith F J, Salkind M R, Jolly B C (1990). Community pharmacy: a method of assessing quality of care. *Soc Sci Med* 31: 603–07.

Smith F J, Jolly B C, Dhillon S (1995). The application of generalisability theory to assessment in a practice-based diploma in clinical pharmacy. *Pharm J* 254: 198–99.

Stevenson M, Taylor J (1995). The effect of a front-shop pharmacist on non-prescription medicine consultations. *J Soc Admin Pharm* 12: 154–58.

Taylor J, Suveges L (1992). Selection of cough, cold and allergy products: the role of consumer-pharmacist interaction. *J Soc Admin Pharm* 9: 59–65.

Williamson V K, Winn S, Livingstone C R, *et al.* (1992). Public views on an extended role for community pharmacy. *Int J Pharm Pract* 1: 223–29.

Wilson M, Robinson E J, Blenkinsopp A, *et al.* (1992). Customers' recall of information given in community pharmacies. *Int J Pharm Pract* 1: 152–59.

3

The reclassification of medicines (I): clinical aspects

Christine Bond

Medicines deregulation

In this section the background to the reclassification of medicines is summarised, together with implications for the profession and the research issues which need addressing.

Background to the reclassification of medicine

Self-medication is a cost-effective component of all healthcare systems, whether they are private or national, and use of standard economic models of supply and demand can show the theoretical economic advantages of switching (Ryan and Bond, 1994). This is summarised in Chapter 4. Until relatively recently the full potential was limited because of legal restrictions on the range of drugs which are available for sale but Government-led moves have increased the number of such drugs by a deregulation process which has been termed 'depomming' by the Medicines Control Agency. This has been supported by both the pharmaceutical profession and the industry but has had a mixed reception from the medical profession (Anonymous, 1992; Spencer and Edwards, 1992). Nonetheless the programme has continued and new deregulations are announced yearly.

A rethinking of the principles on which a medicine's regulatory status is based was prompted by the European Commission in 1987, when it announced its intention to harmonise the distribution of medicines in Europe. The intention was to bring consistency to the availability of medicines, by either prescription or pharmacy sale. For the UK that would have resulted in the ingredients of some pharmacy medicines, such as ephedrine, diphenhydramine, phenylpropanolamine and codeine, moving to prescription-only status. This would have had far-reaching implications for the industry, the NHS and the whole culture of lay care. It was calculated that £100 million sales would have been threatened (Baker, 1993). However, the proposals were reconsidered and approached from the pharmacy perspective, and the decision was that 'no medicine should remain POM unless necessary for reasons of safety'. This became the European Community directive (1992) for medicines classification 92/26/CEE and the basis on which further medicines have been deregulated. The directive stated that medicines should only be POM (Prescription-Only Medicines) if they were:

- dangerous if used other than under medical supervision;
- frequently used incorrectly;
- new and need further investigation;
- normally injected.

The principals of deregulation have also been supported by the World Health Organization in a study of self-medication in Europe, reported by Levin (1998). The conclusions of the study were for 'a framework of orderly development, including reforms in professional education and practice'.

In the US there are currently only two alternative medicine classifications which are 'Prescription Only' or 'General Sale'. There is, however, an ongoing debate around limiting the sale of selected non-prescription medications to pharmacies, which would introduce a third classification for medicines, a similar position to that which exists in the UK. A study by Gore and Thomas (1995) based on a random postal survey of 500 members of the general public – although flawed because of a 49% response rate – showed that stores with pharmacists provided better information to customers on selection and appropriate use of non-prescription medicines, supporting the need for a third category of drugs to be introduced the US. In the meantime, under the current two-category system, it is somewhat surprising that more than 50 prescription drugs have been switched to non-prescription status in the past 20 years (Charupatanapong, 1994). In general the spectrum of medicine available without a prescription is similar to the UK, including the relatively recently available vaginal antifungal treatments. However, proposals to switch salbutamol and topical erythromycin have been blocked. In Australia, salbutamol has been deregulated but there are concerns as to the subsequent control of asthma and there are proposals to recategorise it as a prescription-only medicine (Gibson, 1993).

In 1989 Denmark was amongst the first of the Northern European countries to deregulate a large number of medicines, including cimetidine (Edwards, 1992). Since then other European countries, for example Finland, have also rapidly increased the pace at which medicines are being reclassified. In the period January 1990 to December 1994, 50 products were switched, 19 of them in the preceeding year. Products such as hormone replacement therapy (HRT), haemorrhoid treatments, antihistamines, nicotine replacement therapy (NRT), non-steroidal anti-inflammatory drugs (NSAIDs), and vaginal imidazoles were involved – an interestingly similar list to the UK (Financial Times, 1994).

In contrast, changes have occurred much more slowly in other countries, notably those previously in the Eastern bloc. For example, in Slovakia it is perceived that the Slovak people need more education in self-medication before the Slovak regulations should be allowed to catch up with the legislation of the European Commission. It seems surprising, therefore, that contraceptives and antidepressants feature in a list of expected 'over-the-counter' (OTC) switches.

Thus, across all of Europe and North America, the proposals to deregulate medicines have been quickly implemented.

Reclassification in the UK

The process started slowly in the UK, with the deregulation of ibuprofen and loperamide (1983), terfenadine (1984) and hydrocortisone 1% (topical) (1985) but it has continued steadily with the support of the Government (Bottomley, 1989), the Royal Pharmaceutical Society (Department of Health, 1992, the Council of the Royal Pharmaceutical Society, 1995) and, to a limited extent, the Royal College of General Practitioners (Royal College of General Practitioners, 1993). A list of the recently deregulated or depommed medicines in the UK is shown in Table 3.1.

Future deregulations are inevitable and various lists have been proposed, such as the much quoted list of '51' (Odd, 1992) or the more conservative one included in the consultative document *Pharmaceutical care: the future of community pharmacy* (Department of Health, 1992). This suggested that prescription controls could 'with advantage' be removed from a list of eight products. To date, of these eight, only a compound antibiotic ointment for the treatment of superficial bacterial skin infections, and chloramphenicol 0.5% eye drops for eye infections remain prescription-only medicines. Other target preparations for future deregulations include oral contraceptives and the 'morning after' pill (Anonymous, 1993; Drife, 1993), which has the

Table 3.1 A chronological list of medicines whose UK status has changed from POM (prescription-only medicine) to P (pharmacy-supervised scale) (based on information from the Royal Pharmaceutical Society of Great Britain, 1998)

Date	Ingredient/Product	Date	Ingredient/Product
1983	ibuprofen	1994	diclofenac (topical)
	loperamide		felbinac (topical)
1984	terfenadine		piroxicam (topical)
1985	hydrocortisone 1% (topical)		flunisolide (nasal spray)
1986	miconazole		ranitidine
1988	ibuprofen sr and topical		minoxidil (topical)
1989	astemizole		Adcortyl in Orabase
	mebendazole		Anusol Plus HC ointment
	dextromethorphan		Anusol Plus HC suppositories
1991	nicotine 2 mg gum	1995	hydroxyzine hydrochloride
1992	hyoscine butylbromide		pyrantel embonate
	nicotine patches		fluconazole
	vaginal imidazoles		ketoconazole (shampoo)
	hydrocortisone with crotamiton		hydrocortisone rectal
	(topical)		pseudoephedrine hydrochloride
	carbenoxolone		(extension of exemption)
	paracetamol and dihydrocodeine		cadexomer-iodine
1993	loratidine		budesonide nasal
	aciclovir (topical)		beclomethasone dipropionate
	acrivastine		(extended indications)
	cetirizine	1996	azelastine nasal
	ketoprofen (topical)		nizatidine
	cimetidine		hydrocortisone/lignocaine
	famotidine		hydrochloride spray
	beclomethasone dipropionate		mebeverine hydrochloride
	(nasal)		aciclovir
	mebendazole (multiple dose)	1997	clotrimazole with hydrocortisone
	pseudoephedrine sr	1998	domperidone
	sodium cromoglicate		hydrocortisone and miconazole
	(ophthalmic)		levocabastine
	tioconazole (vaginal)		nedocromil sodium
	nicotine 4 mg gum		ketoconazole cream 2%
	hydrocortisone (oral pellet)		
	aluminium chloride hexahydrate		
	(topical)		

support of both the Royal College of General Practitioners (1995) and the General Medical Services Committee of the British Medical Association (1995).

Regulatory issues

The consensus criteria for deregulation are currently said to be that the drug should be of proven safety, of low toxicity in overdose, and for the treatment of minor 'self-limiting' conditions. The last of these is a vague definition which might already appear to be applied in a less stringent way than was originally envisaged, for example the availability of treatments for vaginal infections. These criteria are applied now, but historically this has not always been the case; aspirin and paracetamol are widely used by the general public, but are not safe in overdose; glyceryl trinitrate tablets and oral theophylline are a further two examples of preparations which have long been available for 'P' (Pharmacy) sale, although they could not be said to be for the treatment of self-limiting conditions; nor are they without side effects (Edwards, 1992). Their 'P' availability is, however, less widely known and the need for doctors to be more aware of this fact has been highlighted to ensure that potentially fatal combinations of over-the-counter and prescribed theophylline are not administered (Thomas, 1986). The rule of a self-limiting condition has not been applied rigorously in Australia, where salbutamol inhalers were made available without a prescription in the early 1980s (Gibson *et al.*, 1993), although, as mentioned earlier, this is currently being reviewed. Interestingly, the change in status of salbutamol inhalers was refused in the UK (Wade, 1991).

The current European position encourages deregulation (see earlier). The UK position is that any new drug entity gaining a medicine licence automatically has POM status. After two years this status defaults to P unless there is a reapplication to retain the POM status. In order to change this POM status subsequently, a formal application has to be made to the MCA. Evidence of safety and efficacy is central to this. The submissions are considered in detail by various Government committees and other relevant professional bodies. It is a time-consuming and expensive process in spite of streamlining of the application procedure (Medicines Control Agency, 1992). It is inevitable, therefore, that if the initiative has come from the industry, as opposed to the professional bodies, subsequent marketing will be used to optimise sales and ensure a viable commercial product and an adequate return on investment. This includes direct advertising to the public, which can lead to problems in practice. The advertising is regulated by the industry under the auspices of the Proprietary Association of Great Britain and standards have recently been raised to come into line with the 1992 European Pharmaceutical Advertising Directive (Proprietary Association of Great Britain, 1994).

Deregulation may be on a brand basis or on an ingredient basis. The latter is the route used by the Royal Pharmaceutical Society when making submissions, for example for the vaginal imidazoles. However, the industry prefers the brand approach, otherwise their investment in the submission would be to the benefit of their competitors. In spite of this, the trend more recently is for the majority of deregulations to be ingredient-based.

Finally, although the net move is towards the deregulation of medicines from POM to P, the status of medicines is constantly under revision Europe-wide (Levin, 1988). There was an outcry from the pharmaceutical profession (Stroh, 1995) when small packs of ibuprofen 200mg (12s) were further reclassified from P to GSL (General Sale List) status (Anonymous, 1995a). This is real deregulation, as almost all restrictions on the sale are then removed, and it is continuing with recent proposals for the GSL status of topical minoxidil for the treatment of male pattern baldness and 2mg nicotine gums. Conversely, carbaryl, a treatment for head lice, has been reversed from P to POM because of evidence of possible carcinogenicity (Anonymous, 1995b); similarly, terfenadine was also reclassified to POM because of serious drug interactions leading to fatal consequences in susceptible individuals (Committee on Safety of Medicines, 1992).

Economic considerations

The theory behind the economic implications of deregulation is explained in full in Chapter 4. However, it is useful to summarise it as follows. Over-the-counter (OTC) purchase of drugs can save patients money as well as time and opportunity costs. Patients are saved the costs of visiting the physician followed by a subsequent visit to the pharmacist. For those patients who would normally pay a prescription charge, the savings will be dependent on the price of the deregulated product. There are already many prescription specialities which are cheaper if bought directly, and a *Drug and Therapeutics* booklet has listed these (1993). This now needs updating. The picture is different if the patient is normally exempt from the prescription charge, and the only savings then are the indirect non-drug costs. If costs are defined to include both monetary and non-monetary elements, it has been shown that the over-the-counter availability of topical 1% hydrocortisone saved patients in the UK £2 million in 1987 alone (Ryan and Yule, 1990).

Savings may also be made by the NHS as drugs become available over the counter. The Government incurs two main costs in the prescribing of a drug; the costs of the physician's time, and the cost of the drug and the payment for its dispensing, whether it be by pharmacist or dispensing doctor. Savings from the depomming of loperamide were estimated to be £3.15 million in 1985, £3.3 million in 1986, and £5 million in 1987 (Ryan and Yule, 1990). The rationale for this is described more fully in Chapter 4.

Finally, the industry has been suffering as a result of the moves to curb NHS spending on drugs. For existing products there is a reduced life after the patent expires, as generic prescribing becomes standard practice (Scottish Medicines Resource Centre, 1993). There is also an increasing need to demonstrate cost effectiveness for new introductions to the list of drugs reimbursed by the NHS (Freemantle *et al.*, 1995); in some countries, such as Australia, this is mandatory. Evidence from the US would certainly indicate that the commercial benefit of switching is very great (Macarthur, 1993). Thus, the industry is looking to the over-the-counter market to extend the brand life of existing products which, contrary to their original fears, does not mean a ban on advertising or cause problems with reimbursement of NHS prescriptions (Hardisty, 1990). Commercial pressure has thus helped speed up depomming but the agenda of the industry is on maximising sales at any cost, and screening for appropriateness by either the GP or the community pharmacist is seen as a barrier to this.

Implications for pharmacy

Whilst many pharmacists welcomed the moves to increase the armamentarium of drugs available for sale under the supervision of a pharmacist, there were also concerns expressed at the responsibility this placed on both pharmacists and their assistants conducting such sales. For example, when the H_2-blockers (H_2-receptor antagonists) were first proposed for deregulation in 1993, both medical and pharmacy representatives highlighted the possible masking of symptoms of serious disease, such as gastric carcinomas, and the prognostic implications resulting from a possible delayed diagnosis. Thus, pharmacists', and their assistants', knowledge base was questioned regarding their ability to appropriately supervise sales, whilst at the same time others were arguing that patients should be free to purchase such newly reclassified drugs without pharmacists taking over the medical paternalistic role.

Indeed, many of the criticisms of the deregulation process were as a result of the involvement of untrained assistants in sales. Yet community pharmacy assistants, as well as community pharmacists, are part of the lay healthcare team, and measures to ensure they have the necessary skills to contribute appropriately are currently being introduced (Stewart, 1994). However, there is little published work on the advice which they give. Krska *et al.* (1994), in a small local study of 16 community pharmacies in Grampian, Scotland, found that assistants were not as likely to give the 'correct' advice when responding to symptoms over the counter. Fisher *et al.* (1991) showed that assistants were less likely to provide concurrent advice when selling over-the-counter medicines. More recently (Ward *et al.*, 1998), it has been shown that assistants themselves are aware of their responsibilities and keen to be part of the pharmacist's team. Indeed, in Chapter 8 of this book, evidence is presented for their important contribution to helping smokers achieve abstinence.

Various proposals and actions have been sought to address the training issues identified above. For example, at one point there was considerable support for the introduction of a 'Super P' drug classification, which would mean that drugs with the new proposed classification would only be able to be sold directly by community pharmacists. Possibilities such as compulsory patient registration with a pharmacist to allow purchase of such products, and record keeping of every such sale were also debated. Although neither of these has materialised, two further developments can, at least in part, be attributed to the concerns about the new 'potent' OTCs (Stewart, 1994). These were the requirement that, by July 1996, all pharmacists' assistants involved in the sale of medicines should hold a qualification the equivalent of NVQ level 2 and, secondly, that all pharmacists should have in their premises a written protocol for the sale of medicines (Anonymous, 1994). This protocol was required to contain information on an exact procedure for ensuring that the pharmacist was aware of all sales, guidance on the questions to be asked of customers before proceeding with a sale, and sometimes specified drugs which, in those premises, only the pharmacist would be allowed to sell.

Whilst the increased range of medicines being made available to the pharmacist for sale as a result of the reclassification were not new, they were new to pharmacists in the context of their proposed use. Thus, there existed in many ways a parallel to the situation in medicine when a totally new medicine is introduced and GPs have to decide when it should be prescribed. Should it be to all patients and would there be some patients who would benefit more than others? In order to disseminate the complex package of information required to answer this range of questions, guidelines were introduced. These are now generally presented in a diagrammatic (algorithmic) version supported by more extensive explanatory text. The guidelines phenomenon has snowballed, with increased emphasis on the need for the contents to be evidence-based, and for the dissemination process to be optimum. In the medical context this has been extensively studied by Grimshaw and Russell (1993).

It was felt that a guideline programme could similarly be of value to pharmacists with the objectives of providing easily accessible, accurate information to support appropriate OTC availability of medicines. The programme of guideline development was system-based and prioritised by recent deregulation. Because of medical concerns, guideline development groups were recommended by the project team (Bond, 1995) to include GPs and pharmacists, relevant hospital consultants, academic pharmacologists and a facilitator.

The research issues

The research questions

The programme of work outlined in the rest of this chapter is a case study of the development of an 'OTC' clinical pharmacy guideline for the treatment of dyspepsia, and an evaluation of its introduction. Thus, it included multidisciplinary development of a clinical guideline for use over the counter in community pharmacies, in the belief that this would provide essential information to pharmacists on newly deregulated products. However, because such initiatives are important, cost money and may be replicated, it is essential that such a programme should be evaluated. This evaluation would need to address the effect of the guideline on pharmacists' knowledge, and a measure of its utility and acceptability in practice, to pharmacists, assistants, and their customers. All three components, the process, the knowledge change, and guideline acceptability, require systematic study.

The research methods

The process of guideline development was in itself innovative, bringing together a range of disciplines and professionals with potentially different attitudes to the recent availability of H_2-blockers over the counter and a lack of familiarity with working with each other. It was considered of value to study this. Research of this type falls within the qualitative domain and uses what are known as case study methodologies.

Typically, these include observation techniques, interviews and focus groups, as well as data extraction from existing documentation such as meeting minutes.

The observational – in this case participant observation – process can be made more objective through the completion of a systematic matrix to record the nature of interactions observed and to relate these to the contributors/meeting members. An example of such a matrix is the Bales and Flanders matrix of interactions (Bales, 1950), previously used by the author in a study of undergraduate medical students (Bond, 1994).

Evaluation of knowledge change resulting from guideline implementation and use requires a different quantitative approach. Research in the medical context has demonstrated the importance of guideline dissemination methods in affecting level of knowledge change. However, there is first a need for preliminary small scale studies which will broadly demonstrate whether or not an improvement in knowledge can be achieved before embarking on large sophisticated study designs involving randomised controlled multi-arm methods. Thus, for a small feasibility study designed merely to indicate the potential of the innovation, a 'before and after' test of knowledge can be used. In order to try and justify associations between any measurable knowledge increase and the guideline, rather than any other incidental causes, such as educational items in the pharmaceutical press, control questions can be introduced into the knowledge test. These are questions which relate to the general topic, in this case disorders of the upper gastrointestinal tract, but are not covered by the guideline per se.

The assessment of the utility and acceptability of the guideline was concerned, in this instance, only with the pharmacist and patient. Pharmacists participating in the study can be asked to monitor their use of the guideline on a prospective basis, known to be better than retrospective methods although still not necessarily reflecting the total picture. (This was discussed in the previous chapters.) In this study, if the form is constructed to collect the required data, it is possible to measure use of the guideline against opportunities for its use and to record reasons why the guideline is not used, such as patient/ client resistance to the structured questioning needed to elucidate the required information.

Finally, in this study, survey methods were used to gain information from pharmacists on their opinions of the guideline.

The studies

In this section there is a description of some of the pilot studies and their results. The small-scale studies are critically discussed and proposals for future work are outlined.

Overview of study design

In order to address the overall research question posed, it was broken down into a series of component questions, as described above, which were answered by an eclectic programme of work. With one exception, individual studies were of a non-experimental research design, allowing study of current activities in their natural social context. That is, on the nomothetic-ideographic continuum (Burrell and Morgan, 1979), the methodologies tend to the ideographic end.

It was necessary to investigate any perceived lack of knowledge and need for training amongst community pharmacists and to formulate and evaluate programmes to meet any identified need. This study of the development of clinical pharmacy guidelines for the treatment of dyspepsia assumed in the planning stage that H_2-blockers would be deregulated, and that, given the widely expressed concern about their appropriate sale from community pharmacies, training would be required. The four-part study was carried out locally for logistical reasons and because location was not considered to be an influential factor on the variables. In summary the study incorporated:

- A small survey of 50 local community pharmacists to assess their perception of the adequacy of their knowledge to take on an extended role, and ways of improving that knowledge.
- The development of a guideline for the treatment of dyspepsia by a multi-disciplinary group which allowed an in-depth observational approach to professional interactions (particularly at the community pharmacy/general practitioner interface) and boundary setting.
- An assessment of the utility of the guideline in daily practice, including patient acceptability.
- An evaluation of the effect of the guideline on knowledge.

Thus, the component parts of this study provided information on the likely uptake of training initiatives by community pharmacists, their perceived value, the potential for interprofessional support and team-working, and the potential for a practical tool which might improve patient outcome and have a concurrent educational benefit. It also gave some small insight into the likely response of the public if a more proactive counselling approach were to be adopted in community pharmacies.

Detailed methods and results

Opinions of community pharmacists

Method   A small questionnaire was designed, piloted and sent to 50 community pharmacists in Aberdeen to assess their attitudes to continuing education, and the role of guidelines. Pharmacists not responding were followed up by telephone reminders.

Results   The questionnaire was sent to all Aberdeen community pharmacies (n = 50). 33 completed questionnaires were returned (a response rate of 66%). The demography of the respondents is shown in Table 3.2.

Thus, the sample reflected the ratio of males and females in the UK but had a higher representation of pharmacists in the younger age group. Other demographic characteristics of the respondents are detailed in Table 3.3.

None of the respondents was a member of the College of Pharmacy Practice, and only one had a postgraduate qualification.

Attitudes to and opinions of continuing education and guidelines   No significant association was found between any of the demographic variables and any attitudinal variable (see Tables 3.4 and 3.5).

Table 3.2 Demography of respondents

Category	Sub-category	Percentage of respondents	UK figures (%)(1990)[a]
Sex	Male	57.6	59.5
	Female	39.4	40.5
	Unspecified	3.0	
Age group	20–24	12.1 }	21.1
	25–29	24.2 }	
	30–34	6.1 }	21.1
	35–39	6.1 }	
	40–44	12.1 }	18.5
	45–49	3.0 }	
	50–54	15.2 }	18.6
	55–59	9.1 }	
	60–64	6.1 }	14.3
	65–69	3.0 }	
	Unspecified	3.0	

[a] Anonymous, 1991.

Table 3.3 Other demographic characteristics

Category	Sub-category	Percentage of respondents
Type of pharmacy	Single handed	45.5
	Small multiple	36.4
	Large multiple	18.1
Type of qualification	BPharm	3
	BSc	60
	PhC	36.4
Place of qualification	Bradford	3
	Edinburgh	3
	Liverpool	3
	Aberdeen	84.8
	Strathclyde	3
	Sunderland	3
Date of first qualification	1950s	30.2
	1960s	6.2
	1970s	21.2
	1980s	24.2
	1990s	18.2
Method of continuing education	Local refresher courses	51.5
	National refresher courses	0
	Other study group	3
	Distance learning	6.1
	Self study	33.3
	Unspecified	6.1
Hours of continuing education in last 12 months	0/unspecified	18.2
	1–10	18.1
	11–20	21.2
	21–30	15.2
	31–40	9.1
	41–50	3
	51–60	9.1
	>60	6.1
	Mean 24.9 hours	

Development of guideline (Bond and Grimshaw, 1995)

Method   After consultation with the gastroenterologists, it was decided to confine the scope of the guidelines to the upper gastrointestinal tract. After an initial literature search, and study of medical models, in particular the North of England Study (Centre for Health Services Research, University of Newcastle, 1991), a multidisciplinary group was convened

Table 3.4 Summary of responses to attitude questions (n = 33)

Statement[a]	Number NO	% NO	Number YES	% YES	Number Don't know	% Don't know
Do you feel that continuing education is essential for a pharmacist to undertake the extended role?	3	9.1	30	90.9		
Do you feel that postgraduate qualifications are essential for the pharmacist to undertake the extended role?	30	90.9	3	9.1		
Do you feel sufficiently knowledgeable to provide safe and appropriate advice when advising patients 'OTC' on the symptoms of minor ailments?	4	12.1	29	87.9		
Do you feel that the further deregulation of medicines (POM to P) will increase the need for pharmacists to be educated regarding response to symptoms?	3	9.1	30	90.9		
Do you ever discuss with your local GP how you should deal with specific symptoms presented 'OTC'?	26	78.8	7	21.2		
Do you feel that your local GP would be interested in helping you to develop agreed methods (treatment protocols) of dealing with 'OTC' advice about minor ailments?	16	48.5	14	42.4	3	9.1

[a] The respondents were asked for a YES/NO answer to the following statements.

Table 3.5 Summary of responses to questions on protocol development (n = 33)

Statement[a]	Number (%) strongly agree 1	Number (%) agree 2	Number (%) uncertain 3	Number (%) disagree 4	Number (%) strongly disagree 5	Number (%) Don't know	Mean
The development of agreed treatment protocols would be a useful educative exercise for community pharmacists.	10 (30.3)	13 (39.4)	4 (12.1)	4 (12.1)	2 (6.1)		2.24
The development of agreed treatment protocols would be useful in developing interprofessional collaboration.	9 (27.3)	10 (30.3)	9 (27.3)	1 (3)	4 (12.1)		2.42
Using agreed protocols would be a useful educative exercise for community pharmacists.	6 (18.2)	17 (51.5)	6 (18.2)	1 (3)	3 (9.1)		2.33
I would be interested in taking part in an exercise to develop agreed protocols.	6 (18.2)	7 (21.2)	14 (42.4)	2 (6.1)	3 (9.1)	1 (3)	2.58
I would be interested in using agreed protocols developed by others on a pilot basis.	7 (21.2)	14 (42.4)	5 (15.2)	1 (3)	3 (9.1)	3 (9.1)	2.09

a The respondents were asked to circle on a scale of 1–5 (strongly agree to strongly disagree) their level of agreement with the following statements.

to develop the guideline. All potential local stakeholders were identified and representatives were invited to participate in the multiprofessional group, which consisted of two community pharmacists, two general practitioners, a gastroenterologist, a clinical pharmacist (academic), a group leader, a research assistant and a facilitator. The facilitator was skilled in the development and implementation of medical guidelines, and had been previously involved in the development of hospital out-patient referral guidelines in the same clinical area. The general practitioners were nominated by a local professional committee (the General Practice Subcommittee of the Area Medical Committee), likewise the community pharmacists were nominated by the Area Pharmaceutical Committee. The academic clinical pharmacist specialised in gastro-enterology.

The group met five times during December, January and early February, and developed an algorithmic guideline and supporting documentation. A case study approach was used to follow this development, primarily based on observation, substantiated by an adaptation of the Bales and Flanders matrix of interactions (Bales, 1950). Definition of the interaction classifications is shown in Figure 3.1.

Results   The following description of the five development meetings is based on the detailed notes taken at each meeting and the author's observations, combined with the interactions analysis.

Proposing	A behaviour which puts forward a new concept, suggestion or course of action
Supporting	A behaviour which involves a conscious and direct declaration of support or agreement with another person or his concepts
Disagreeing	A behaviour which involves a conscious and direct declaration of difference of opinion or criticism of another person or his concepts
Giving information	A behaviour which offers facts, opinions or clarification to other individuals
Seeking information	A behaviour which seeks facts, opinions, or clarification from another individual or individuals
Building	A behaviour which extends or develops a proposal which has been made by another person

Figure 3.1 The Bales and Flanders matrix of interactions: explanation of categories

First and second meetings Due to constraints imposed by the project timetable and different availabilities of group members, the first and second meetings were conducted without the gastroenterologist. It was realised that this would have implications for subsequent meetings but it was unfortunately unavoidable. Otherwise all professions were represented. The issues addressed in the first meeting included defining the tasks of the group, dealing with professional hierarchies and personalities, developing both interprofessional mutual respect and understanding of different professionals' working environments and experiences of managing patients with dyspepsia. Little progress was made towards the actual guideline, which concerned some group members. The second meeting was more productive and there was a positive atmosphere reflecting the importance of the initial small group work during the first meeting. During the meeting the group began to develop the guideline using an algorithmic structure. The group defined the condition and patient groups covered by the guideline and identified important presenting symptoms where immediate referral to a general practitioner was felt to be indicated (e.g. persistent vomiting, haematemesis, melaena, weight loss, dysphagia, jaundice).

Third meeting The facilitator was unable to attend this meeting. It was the first meeting which the gastroenterologist was able to attend, and in many respects duplicated much of the group work of the first meeting as the consultant had to acquire an understanding of the task. There was a re-emergence of issues relating to professional hierarchies and areas of professional responsibilities between both secondary and primary care and primary and pharmaceutical/self care. Since the consultant's knowledge of community pharmacy was more limited than the general practitioners', the task of establishing mutual professional understanding and respect was more difficult. There was a definite feeling of 'two steps forward and three steps back'. Little progress was made in developing the guideline; exclusions to treatment were extended and treatment options were restricted to short courses of antacids.

Fourth meeting and fifth meeting The fourth meeting was much more productive, most of the ground lost at the third meeting was made up. The discussion often reflected participants' differing perspectives and perceptions of the condition, but the participants were ready to work towards a consensus. The algorithm progressed through all the treatment stages, and included guidelines for when cimetidine could safely and appropriately be recommended by community pharmacists. The need for detailed documentation to accompany the guideline was also identified. The guideline was finalised at the fifth meeting, the branching logic of the guideline was rechecked, the wording of the accompanying documentation was discussed and any outstanding inconsistencies were addressed. The format of the final guidance is shown in Figure 3.2 (Bond and Grimshaw, 1994).

Small group work during guideline development The meetings were conducted in a generally positive fashion, with an increasingly relaxed atmosphere. As the meetings progressed we noted less professional segregation in the seating arrangements. The atmosphere at the meetings became more relaxed, jokes were made and there was an increasing tendency for informal interprofessional discussion before and after the meetings, not necessarily related to the matter in hand.

Most interactions were proposing or supporting new ideas, confirming the positive atmosphere of the meetings (with the exception of the third meeting where there were higher levels of disagreement). This was particularly pronounced in the fourth and fifth meetings as the group finalised the guideline. Similarly, total interactions increased at these later meetings, although meeting length remained fairly constant at around one hour. This is shown in Table 3.6, using the Bales and Flanders categories.

The relative input of the different professions appears to reflect professional hierarchies, although individual personalities will inevitably have some bearing on this. In spite of his attending only three of the five meetings, most input was made by the gastoenterologist, followed by the group leader. Of the two community pharmacists, one contributed almost twice as much as the other, illustrating the

Table 3.6 Results from Bales and Flanders analysis: summary of interactions by meeting. (Reproduced with permission from Bond and Grimshaw, 1995.)

Interaction	Meeting 1	Meeting 2	Meeting 3	Meeting 4	Meeting 5	Totals
Proposing new concepts	4	4	7	12	13	40
Supporting	5	9	8	8	5	35
Disagreeing	6	2	7	1	3	19
Giving information	6	8	7	7	10	38
Seeking information	2	2	7	5	5	21
Building	5	3	2	2	4	16
Totals	28	28	38	35	40	169

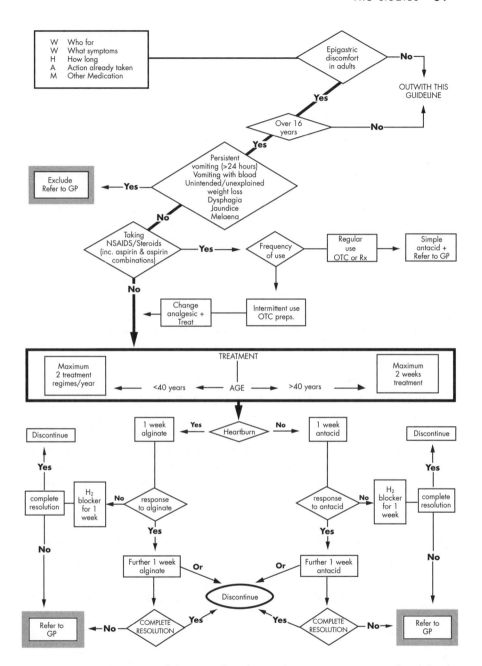

Figure 3.2 Dyspepsia guideline (Bond and Grimshaw, 1994). Reprinted with kind permission of the *Pharmaceutical Journal*.

influence of personality; the contributions from the two general practitioners were more similar. A summary of these issues is detailed in Figure 3.3.

Pilot of guideline utility

An overview of the design is shown in Figure 3.4.

Method Ten local Aberdeen pharmacies were identified to pilot the guideline for utility and ease of use. At the same time, the two community pharmacists who were part of the development group also assessed the guideline from a practical viewpoint. As the deregulation of the H_2-blockers was at that time announced but not yet legislated for (Anonymous, 1994), a version of the guideline was prepared for the pilot study which excluded the H_2-blockers. The pilot study was carried out for a one-month period in late March and early April 1993. The members of the guideline development group representing the professional bodies (Area Pharmaceutical Committee and the General Practice subcommittee of the Area Medical Committee) also reported back to their parent bodies.

As a result of this final consultative stage, there were no significant amendments and a full pilot was implemented. All Grampian community pharmacists (n = 124) together with community pharmacists in the Inverness area (n = 10) were invited to participate in a pilot study of the guideline's utility. Those unable to attend one of the launch meetings were either visited personally or the guideline and information were sent by post. The latter was the least favoured mechanism for dissemination

---

- Problems of professional hierarchies between pharmacists and medical colleagues.
- Problems of professional hierarchies between primary and secondary care.
- Medical colleagues' ignorance of pharmacists' education.
- Medical colleagues' ignorance of pharmacists' working practice.
- Shortcomings of pharmacists' current working environment.
- Resistance to change.

Figure 3.3 Protocol development meetings: problems encountered and issues raised

because medical studies have demonstrated that guidelines are most successfully implemented after face-to-face meetings (Grimshaw and
Russell, 1993).

At the meetings there was an initial test of knowledge of the gastrointestinal tract (the GIST: see below), the development and rationale of
the guidelines was explained and the documentation for the study of
guideline utility was presented. There was opportunity for questions and
a multidisciplinary discussion of common problems.

Community pharmacists were asked to use the guideline every time
they were requested to provide advice on symptoms of the upper gastrointestinal tract over a period of three months; each such advice contact

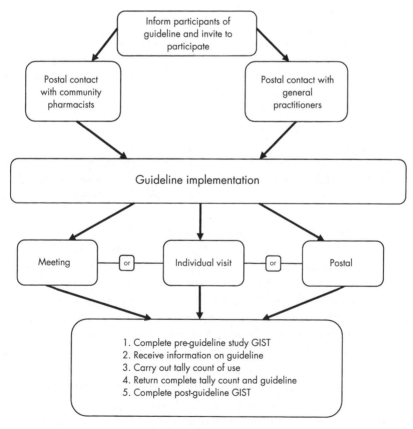

Figure 3.4 Utility of guideline: study design

was noted on a tally chart. Community pharmacists were also asked to note similar advice contacts where, for whatever reason, they had been unable to use the guideline. They were also asked to note the number of direct sales of products for the treatment of dyspepsia when no advice was involved.

At the end of the three-month pilot period, participating community pharmacists were asked to return the guideline pack, supporting information and tally counts of use. On receipt of the returned guideline documentation the community pharmacists were finally asked to complete a Guideline Evaluation Questionnaire which asked about ease of use, acceptability to pharmacist, acceptability to patient, modification in practice, interest in future guidelines on other topics, and a second test of knowledge of the gastrointestinal tract (GIST).

Results   The recruitment and response of the community pharmacists is shown in Table 3.7, and the frequency of the guideline use are in Table 3.8.

Three pharmacists recorded no dyspepsia advice contacts either using or not using the guideline. All records on their tally charts were for direct sales. t-tests for independent samples demonstrated that pharmacists who attended dissemination meetings used the guideline more than pharmacists who did not attend a meeting (t = 0.026, 95% confidence intervals). The responses to the detailed evaluation of guideline utility are shown in Table 3.9.

Chi-square tests of association demonstrated that pharmacists who attended dissemination meetings found the guideline easier to use (Chi Square 4.85; df = 1; p = 0.028, Yates corrected; Fisher's exact test p = 0.015).

No other statistically significant correlations were noted.

In summary, the subjective evaluation of the guideline as measured by the postal questionnaire was overwhelmingly supportive. Respondents found both the guideline and explanatory notes useful, and agreed with the information. Most community pharmacists found the guideline easy to use and preferred the diagrammatic version. Those who had attended the dissemination meetings or who had had a face-to-face visit from a member of the research team were significantly more likely to find the guideline easy to use and had used it more frequently. 40% of respondents found that sometimes patients were not responsive to such structured questioning. All but one pharmacist requested a copy of the guideline to keep and all but one requested guidelines for other therapeutic areas.

Table 3.7 Recruitment and response of community pharmacists

Number of community pharmacists attending guideline dissemination meetings	16
Number of community pharmacists recruited by postal dissemination	13
Number of community pharmacists recruited by individual contact	10
Total recruitment	39

3 community pharmacists withdrew for ill health
3 community pharmacists moved

Final sample size[a]	33
Number completed tally counts	29 (88%)
Number completed evaluations	32 (97%)
Number completed 'after' GISTS	23 (70%)

[a] Reasons for dropout: withdrew from study (no tally count or GIST) 4; did not do 'after' GIST ('forgot', 'no time',) 4; 'after' GIST lost in post 2.

Table 3.8 Details of frequency of guideline use per week

Guideline use	Frequency per week	Range per 3 months
Average number of times guideline used	1.97	0–69
Average number of times guideline not used	1.28	0–59
Average total dyspepsia contacts	3.25	
NOTE: Average number direct 'non-advice' sales	2.67	0–287

Evaluation of knowledge

Method A gastrointestinal knowledge assessment form (GIST) was developed and included general questions on the gastrointestinal tract together with additional questions reflecting the content of the guideline. Pharmacists completed the assessment before and after the trial use of the guideline. Thus, each community pharmacist acted as his/her own control. Identification of individual forms was voluntary, so that pharmacists would not feel intimidated.

Table 3.9 Responses to evaluation of guideline utility questionnaire (n = 32)

Question	YES (percentage)	NO (percentage)	Don't know (percentage)
Did you find the diagrammatic guideline useful?	31 (97)	1 (3)	0 (0)
Did you find the explanatory notes useful?	31 (97)	1 (3)	0 (0)
Did you agree with the information given in the diagram and explanatory notes?	31 (97)	0 (0)	1 (3)
Was the diagrammatic guideline easy to use in practice?	21 (66)	10 (31)	1 (3)
Were the patients responsive to structured questioning?	14 (44)	11 (34)	7 (22)
Did you have to ask any further questions not suggested by the guideline?	7 (22)	24 (75)	1 (3)
Did you tailor the diagrammatic guideline to your own needs?	17 (53)	15 (47)	0 (0)
Considering only the presentation of the guideline did you prefer the diagram (YES) or explanatory notes (NO)?	22 (69)	10 (31)	0 (0)
Do you have any recommendations for improving the guideline?	16 (50)	14 (44)	2 (6)
Would you be interested in receiving a copy of the revised guideline?	31 (97)	1 (3)	0 (0)
Would you be interested in receiving guidelines covering other therapeutic topics?	28 (88)	1 (3)	3 (9)

Results   Of the sample of 33 community pharmacists only 23 (70%) completed both before and after GIST and only 17 paired sets of data were available for analysis, due to anonymity of some of the forms. Forms were marked in two ways. First, questions were either marked as right or wrong; additionally, questions were allocated a mark dependent on the number of possible answer components. This allowed more credit to be given for partially correct answers. Detailed results of the before and after test are shown below in Tables 3.10 and 3.11, which are based on 36 pre-study GISTs and 23 post-study GISTs. The data are therefore unpaired. There was an overall increase in knowledge of the gastro-intestinal tract over the study period. However, when guideline-related and non-guideline-related questions were separated, there was 24.36% improvement in guideline-related questions and 10.59% improvement in non-guideline-related questions.

The analyses were repeated using the 17 paired data sets. The results on the basis of numbers of questions right and wrong are shown in Tables 12 and 13. This indicated an average of 11.9% improvement in the guideline-related questions and 0.92% in the non-guideline-related questions.

The distributions of the exact test marks for GIST-related and non-GIST-related questions before and after pilot use of the guideline were plotted and inspected. As the frequencies of the exact marks did not follow a normal distribution, the means of these exact test marks were compared using a non-parametric test for paired samples (the Wilcoxon matched pairs, signed ranks test). The results are shown in Table 3.14.

Thus, there was evidence to demonstrate a significant increase in knowledge in the GIST-related questions which could be attributed to

Table 3.10 Summary of percentage guideline-related questions completed correctly before and after use of guideline (unpaired data)

GIST scores: guideline-related questions

Question	% right before	% wrong before	% unsure before	% right after	% wrong after	% unsure after	Difference in % right
1	50	7.1	42.9	82.6	4.3	13	32.6
2	53.6	3.6	42.9	91.3	0	8.7	37.7
3	60.7	25	14.3	73.9	0	26.1	13.2
5	57.1	17.9	25	87	13	0	29.9
6a	67.9	17.9	14.3	82.6	13	4.3	14.7
6b	35.7	42.9	21.4	60.9	13	26.1	25.2
9	42.9	14.3	42.9	78.3	4.3	17.4	35.4
10	35.7	25	39.3	60.9	8.7	30.4	25.2
18	57.1	7.1	35.7	65.2	4.3	30.4	8.1
19	39.3	21.4	39.3	60.9	13	26	21.6
						Total	243.6
				Average difference per question			24.36

Table 3.11 Summary of percentage non-guideline-related questions completed correctly before and after use of guideline (unpaired data)

GIST scores: non-guideline-related questions

Question	% right before	% wrong before	% unsure before	% right after	% wrong after	% unsure after	Difference in % right
4a	39.3	60.7	0	43.5	56.5	0	4.2
4b	28.6	71.4	0	34.8	65.2	0	6.2
4c	46.4	53.6	0	43.5	56.5	0	−2.9
4d	75	25	0	78.3	21.7	0	3.3
4e	100	0	0	100	0	0	0
4f	82.1	17.9	0	95.7	4.3	0	13.6
4g	75	25	0	65.2	34.8	0	−9.8
7	50	7.1	42	95.7	0	4.3	45.7
8	53.6	21.4	25	69.6	4.3	26.1	16
11a	71.4	28.6	0	73.9	26.1	0	2.5
11b	89.3	10.7	0	87	13	0	−2.3
11c	92.9	7.1	0	100	0	0	7.1
11d	64.3	35.7	0	69.6	30.4	0	5.3
11e	82.1	17.9	0	91.3	8.7	0	9.2
12	21.4	10.7	67.9	69.6	4.3	26.1	48.2
13	14.3	14.3	71.4	4.3	0	95.7	−10
14	42.9	3.6	53.6	65.2	4.3	30.4	22.3
15	85.7	0	14.3	95.7	0	4.3	10
16a	92.9	7.1	0	100	0	0	7.1
16b	78.6	21.4	0	65.2	34.8	0	−13.4
17	78.6	0	21.4	95.7	4.3	0	17.1
20a	46.4	0	53.6	65.2	4.3	30.4	18.8
20b	92.9	0	7.1	100	0	0	7.1
20c	25	35.7	39.3	73.9	8.7	17.4	48.9
						Total	254.2
				Average difference per question			10.59

the guideline. Only very small differences were noted for the non-guideline-related questions which were not statistically significant. There were also indications that the more knowledgeable participants were more likely to complete the follow-up GISTs and to identify their forms.

Limitations and implications

Study limitations

This study was small and had some limitations which are now briefly discussed. The participants were self-selected and from a discrete

Table 3.12 Summary of percentage guideline-related questions completed correctly before and after use of guideline (paired data only)

GIST scores: guideline-related questions

Question	% right before	% wrong before	% unsure before	% right after	% wrong after	% unsure after	Difference in % right
1	29.4	5.9	64.7	29	12	59	0
2	29.4	70.6	0	35	6	59	6
3	35.3	52.9	11.8	65	12	24	30
5	76.5	11.8	11.8	82	0	18	6
6a	11.8	76.5	11.8	47	41	12	35
6b	11.8	70.6	17.6	29	53	18	17
9	76.5	11.8	11.8	76	12	12	0
10	76.5	76.5	11.8	41	24	35	−35
18	23.5	23.5	52.9	53	12	5	30
19	23.5	29.4	47.1	53	18	29	30
						Total	119
				Average difference per question			11.9

geographical area, raising questions about their representativeness compared to the wider population of community pharmacists. Although there was evidence to suggest that they were similar in terms of sex, there was a higher representation of younger pharmacists, and there could, for example, have been base-line knowledge differences. The response rate to the follow-up knowledge test was also disappointingly low and this raises further questions about the generalisability of the knowledge improvement demonstrated. In this pilot study, a range of dissemination methods was used because of the pragmatic nature of the work. This included group meetings, one-to-one educational outreach and mailed information. The relative numbers in each category are shown in Table 3.7. Thus, the intervention was not strictly homogeneous, and the pharmacists themselves also self-selected into the various methods. The best method of dissemination of the guideline also has to be considered. The small numbers make proper comparisons difficult, but a trend was noted which indicated that pharmacists attending meetings face to face either at a group meeting or on an individual basis, said they found the guideline easier to use and used it more frequently. Finally, the study did not attempt to evaluate the impact of the guideline on the outcomes of care, and only considered self-reported changes in the process of care. Nonetheless, the study did have some important and valid pointers for future practice and research.

A summary of the key study findings is shown in Figure 3.5.

Table 3.13 Summary of percentage non-guideline-related questions completed correctly before and after use of guideline (paired data)

GIST scores: non-guideline-related questions

Question	% right before	% wrong before	% unsure before	% right after	% wrong after	% unsure after	Difference in % right
4a	35.3	58.8	5.9	41	53	6	5
4b	41.2	58.8	0	47	53	0	6
4c	41.2	58.8	0	47	53	0	6
4d	70.6	29.4	0	76	24	0	5
4e	100	0	0	100	0	0	0
4f	82.4	17.6	0	94	6	0	11
4g	70.6	29.4	0	71	29	0	0
7	70.6	29.4	0	76	24	0	5
8	70.6	29.4	0	82	12	6	11
11a	76.5	23.5	0	71	29	0	−5
11b	82.4	17.6	0	76	24	0	−6
11c	94.1	5.9	0	100	0	0	6
11d	64.7	35.3	0	65	35	0	0
11e	82.4	17.6	0	94	6	0	12
12	41.2	29.4	29.4	24	29	47	−17
13	41.2	52.9	5.9	35	65	0	−6
14	41.2	5.9	52.9	53	0	47	12
15	88.2	11.8	0	82	0	18	−6
16a	88.2	11.8	0	100	0	0	12
16b	76.5	23.5	0	59	41	0	−17
17	88.2	11.8	0	94	0	6	6
20a	35.3	5.9	58.8	35	0	65	0
20b	100	0	0	94	6	0	−6
20c	11.8	64.7	23.5	6	65	29	−6
						Total	22
					Average difference per question		0.92

Implications for the future

The work detailed in the earlier part of this section has provided clear evidence for the feasibility of and benefit of OTC clinical guidelines in community pharmacies. The study does, however, leave many questions unanswered, such as the generalisability of the findings to other conditions, and to larger groups of pharmacists and their assistants.

Future work should include much larger numbers of community pharmacists, randomly allocated to the range of educational methods

Table 3.14 Wilcoxon matched pairs, signed ranks test on guideline-related and non-guideline-related questions. (Reproduced with permission from Bond *et al.*, 1998.)

Question type	Time of test	Mean test score	z value	2-tail p
Guideline-related	Before	9.1	−3.6214	0.0003
Guideline-related	After	12		
Non-guideline-related	Before	24.47	−0.9021	0.3670
Non-guideline-related	After	24.74		

- Aberdeen community pharmacists were confident of their current ability to treat symptoms of minor ailments, but were favourably disposed to using clinical pharmacy guidelines and participating in continuing education.
- A multidisciplinary group representing various members of the medical and pharmaceutical professions successfully developed a guideline for the treatment of dyspepsia.
- Observation of the development group allowed exploration of other interprofessional issues.
- The vast majority of community pharmacists found the guideline practical and useful and would like guidelines for other areas.
- Knowledge of the treatment of dyspepsia was improved significantly in those community pharmacists using the guideline.

Figure 3.5 Summary of findings

tested above to demonstrate clearly the relative benefit of each. Evaluation of such a study should include a health economic component as, in NHS terms, the 'best method' will be the most cost effective method. Another factor not addressed by the small-scale studies described here is observed effect of guidelines on practice, as mentioned under the study limitations. As a result of the dissemination of best practice, do pharmacists actually behave differently? Is the process of care altered, and if so what is the effect on patient outcome? Are patients more likely to receive the best treatment, are patients with symptoms of more significant disease referred more quickly for medical advice, and do patients receiving 'best' OTC treatment improve any more quickly?

Additionally, from the patients' perspective, what do they think about the role of the pharmacist in having a more interventionist paternalistic role (Prayle and Brazier, 1998)? As the range of deregulated medicines increases and products are used by wider and more varied populations, what do we know about the safety of medicines in this context? Should all sales be recorded? If the NHS net finally, as is strongly recommended, includes community pharmacists, should GPs be routinely notified of all such sales, and if so is this an infringement of a patient's civil liberty?

Thus, the small studies reported in this chapter have merely provided a flavour of the benefit of guidelines and of their contribution to the success of the initiative to make more medicines available without a prescription. With the reconfigured NHS (Department of Health (1997), Secretary of State for Scotland (1997)), the evolving of Primary Care Groups (PCGs) and Local Health Care Cooperatives (LHCCs) in Scotland and pharmacists' involvement in these, both based in medical premises and from the traditional 'high street' base, the potential for agreed local strategies in the treatment of minor illnesses is enhanced. The pharmacists' guidelines should be coherent with any medical guidelines available for the same therapeutic area so that seamless care across the community (self-care) and primary care interface is provided and common messages are given to avoid public confusion and reinforce good and appropriate advice-seeking behaviour.

Acknowledgements

Crown copyright material is reproduced with the permission of the Queen's Printer for Scotland.

We would like to acknowledge the contribution of all healthcare professionals and patients to these studies. We also acknowledge the funding provided by the Pharmacy Practice Research Fund, Scottish Office Home and Health Department. Work reported in this chapter was originally published as original research (Bond and Grimshaw, 1995 and Bond et al., 1998).

References

Anonymous (1992). Royal College of GPs accepts pharmacy report with reservations. *Pharm J* 249: 305.
Anonymous (1993). Editorial. Ocs o-t-c? *Lancet* 342: 565–566.
Anonymous (1994). Protocols and staff training to be added to Code of Ethics. *Pharm J* 252: 124.
Anonymous (1995a). GSL Ibuprofen product to be marketed this month. *Pharm J* 254: 12.

Anonymous (1995b). POM-to-P shift proposed for budesonide and P-to-POM for carbaryl. *Pharm J* 255: 138.

Baker M (1993). POM to P: Who controls? *Proceedings of members meeting July 1993*. London: Proprietary Association of Great Britain.

Bales R F (1950). *Interaction process analysis: a method for the study of small groups*. Cambridge, Mass: Addison-Wesley.

Bond C M (1994). *Teaching in the undergraduate medical curriculum: a study of the effect of gender and other factors*. MEd Thesis. University of Aberdeen.

Bond C M (1995). *Prescribing in community pharmacy: barriers and opportunities*. PhD Thesis. University of Aberdeen.

Bond C M, Grimshaw J M (1994). Clinical guidelines for the treatment of dyspepsia in community pharmacies. *Pharm J* 252: 228.

Bond C M, Grimshaw J M (1995). Multidisciplinary guideline development: a case study from community pharmacy. *Health Bulletin* 53: 26–33.

Bond C M, Grimshaw J M, Taylor R *et al.* (1998). The evaluation of clinical guidelines to ensure appropriate 'over-the-counter' advice in community pharmacies. *Journal of Social and Administrative Pharmacy* 15: 33–9.

Bottomley V (1989). Reported in POM to P call to meet government's health challenge. *Pharm J* 243: 728.

Burrell G, Morgan G (1979). *Sociological paradigms and organisational analysis*. London: Heinemann.

Centre for Health Services Research, University of Newcastle (1991). *North of England study of standards and performance in general practice*. Report 50.

Charupatanapong N (1994). Perceived likelihood of risks in self medication practices. *J Soc Admin Pharm* 11(1): 18–27.

Committee on Safety of Medicines and Medicines Control Agency (1992). *Astemizole and terfenadine. Current problems in Pharmacovigilance*: 35.

Council of the Royal Pharmaceutical Society of Great Britain (1995). *Annual Report*. London: Pharmaceutical Press.

Department of Health (1997). *The New NHS – Modern and dependable*.

Department of Health and Royal Pharmaceutical Society of Great Britain (1992). *Pharmaceutical Care: the future for community pharmacy*. London: Royal Pharmaceutical Society of Great Britain.

Drife J O (1993). Deregulating emergency contraception. *BMJ* 307: 695–96.

Drug and Therapeutics Bulletin (1993). Medicines cheaper over the counter. *Drug Ther Bull* 31(15): supplement.

Edwards C (1992). Liberalising medicines supply. *Int J Pharm Pract* 1(4): 186.

European Community (1992). *Directive for medicines classification*. 92/26/EEC.

Financial Times (1994). *Finland steps up pace of switching*. OTC Business News November 24: 9,10,13.

Fisher C M, Corrigan O I, Henman M C (1991). A study of community pharmacy practice. 3. Non-prescribed medicines sales and counselling. *J Soc Admin Pharm* 8(2): 69–75.

Freemantle N, Henry D, Maynard A, *et al.* (1995). Promoting cost effective prescribing: Britain lags behind. *BMJ* 310: 955–56.

General Medical Services Committee (1995). Reported in More support for OTC emergency contraception. *Pharm J* 254: 572.

Gibson P, Henry D, Francis L, *et al.* (1993). Association between non prescription beta 2 agonist inhalers and under treatment of asthma. *BMJ* 306: 1514–18.

Gore M R, Thomas J (1995). Non-prescription information services in pharmacies and alternative stores: implications for a third class of drugs. *J Soc Admin Pharm* 12(2): 86–99.

Grimshaw J M, Russell I T (1993). Effect of clinical guidelines on medical practice: a systematic review of rigorous evaluations. *Lancet* 342: 1317–22.

Hardisty B (1990). The enigma of OTC advertising. *Pharm J* 245: 321.

Krska J, Greenwood R, Howitt E P (1994). Audit of advice provided in response to symptoms. *Pharm J* 252: 93–96.

Levin L S (1988). Self medication in Europe: some perspectives on the role of the pharmacist. In: Lund L, Dukes G, eds. *The role and function of the pharmacist in Europe*. Report of a WHO working group. Groningen: Styx Publications.

Macarthur D (1993). *OTC switches – hope or hype?* Dorking: Donald Macarthur.

Medicines Control Agency (1992). *Changing the legal classification of a prescription only medicine for human use*. MAL 77. London: MCA.

Odd R (1992). *Proceedings of Medicines Control Agency POM to P seminar*. London: Royal Pharmaceutical Society of Great Britain.

Prayle D, Brazier M (1998). Supply of medicines: paternalism, autonomy and reality. *J Med Ethics* 24: 93–98.

Proprietary Association of Great Britain (1994). *Code of standards of advertising practice for over-the-counter medicines*. London: PAGB.

Royal College of General Practitioners (1993). Comment by the Royal College of General Practitioners on the Report of the Joint Working Party on the future role of the Community Pharmaceutical Services. *Royal College of General Practitioners 1993 Members' Reference Book* 145–149. London: RCGP.

Royal College of General Practitioners (1995). Reported in RCGP votes for emergency contraception OTC. *Pharm J* 254: 185.

Royal Pharmaceutical Society of Great Britain (1998). *Bibliography. Prescription only medicines reclassified to pharmacy only medicines*. London: RPSGB.

Ryan M, Bond C M (1996). Using the economic theory of consumer surplus to estimate the benefits of dispensing doctors and prescribing pharmacists. *J Soc Admin Pharm* 13(4): 178–87.

Ryan M, Yule B (1990). Switching drugs from prescription-only to over-the-counter availability: economic benefits in the United Kingdom. *Health Policy* 16: 233–39.

Scottish Medicines Resource Centre (1993). Generic prescribing. *Medicines Resource* 10: 358.

Secretary of state for Scotland (1997). *Designed to care: renewing the National Health Service in Scotland.*

Spencer J, Edwards C (1992). Pharmacy beyond the dispensary: general practitioners' views. *BMJ* 304: 1670–72.

Stewart A (1994). Staff training: fountain of knowledge or a mirage. *Pharm J* 253: 728.

Stroh B (1995). Medicines classification. *Pharm J* 255: 167.

Thomas C E (1986). Over-the-counter theophyllines. *J R Coll Gen Pract* 3(6): 180.

Wade A (1991). Personal communication. London: Science Committee, Royal Pharmaceutical Society of Great Britain.

Ward P R, Bissell P, Noyce P R (1998). Medicines counter assistants: roles and responsibilities in the sale of deregulated medicines. *Int J Pharm Pract* 6(4): 207–15.

4

The reclassification of medicines (II): economic aspects

Mandy Ryan

Introduction

This chapter looks at the contribution health economics can make to the debate on extending the role of pharmacists in the provision of drugs. Central to the discipline of economics are the concepts of 'scarcity', 'choice' and 'opportunity cost'. Resources are 'scarce', thus, every time we 'choose' to use them in one way we give up the 'opportunity' of using them in other ways. Thus, the implication of scarcity, choice and opportunity cost is that decisions have to be made concerning the most efficient way to provide healthcare resources. Within the context of the reclassification of drugs, this means deciding what is the most efficient way to provide drugs. Economics can be seen as a framework to assist in answering this question. It does this by attempting to identify, measure and value the costs and benefits of alternative systems for providing drugs. Economics is a decision-aiding instrument for the allocation of society's scarce healthcare resources. This chapter outlines the various benefits and costs relevant to the debate concerning the reclassification of medicines.

Identifying and measuring costs and benefits when reclassifying drugs

The economic concept of cost is 'opportunity cost'. This concept takes as it starting point the premise that resources are scarce. Therefore, every time we choose to use resources in one way, we are giving up the 'opportunity' of using them in other beneficial activities. The opportunity cost of any healthcare intervention is therefore defined as the benefit forgone from not using that resource in its best alternative use. Only if a resource has a next best use does it have an opportunity cost. The concept of opportunity cost also embodies the crucial notion of sacrifice – in economics something only has 'value' if a sacrifice has been made, or is being made for it.

Using this definition of cost, items to be included on the cost side of an economic evaluation are any 'resources' which have an alternative use. Often, costs (and benefits) are mis-classified within economic evaluations (Donaldson and Shackley, 1997). For example, anxiety has often been counted as a 'cost' and cost savings as 'benefits'. However, anxiety per se does not have an 'opportunity cost'; it is not a resource which could be used in some other activity. Anxiety is a negative effect on health or well-being and should be accounted for on the benefit side of an evaluation. Likewise, 'cost savings' are negative costs and should be accounted for on the cost side.

Up until the early 1990s benefit assessment in health economics focused almost exclusively on health outcomes (Williams, 1985; EuroQol, 1990; Kind et al., 1994). During the 1990s some health economists argued that benefit assessment should extend beyond health outcomes and take account of non-health outcomes and process attributes (Gerard et al., 1992; Mooney and Lange, 1993; Mooney, 1994; Ryan, 1995; Donaldson et al., 1995). Non-health outcomes refer to sources of benefit such as the provision of information, reassurance, anxiety, autonomy and dignity in the provision of care. Process attributes include such aspects of care as travelling time, waiting time, staff seen, location of treatment, continuity of care, and staff attitudes.

Given the above definition of costs and benefits, Table 4.1 provides a summary of the costs and benefits to be considered when switching drugs from prescription-only to over-the-counter (OTC) availability.

Identifying and measuring costs

Staffing costs include the costs of any medical personnel involved in the delivery of healthcare. In the case of the reclassification of drugs this may involve the time of doctors, nurses, pharmacists and pharmacy assistants. There will only be an opportunity cost of staff time if time released could be used in an alternative way (Ratcliffe et al., 1996). When the drug is 'obtained' from the doctor (ie. on a NHS reimbursable prescription), staffing costs are incurred. Assuming that the doctor's time has an opportunity cost, the value of this time may be proxied by their salary. If the drug is obtained directly from the pharmacist without a prescription, the remuneration to the pharmacist is simply the profit on the drug. Thus, there are no costs to the NHS of a patient obtaining drugs OTC.

Table 4.1 Potential costs and benefits of reclassifying medicines

Resource use/costs	*(Dis)Benefits to society*
National Health Service Staffing costs Consumables	**Changes in health**

Patients and their families
Change in cost of drugs
Reduced travelling expenses
Reduced time lost from other
  activities (i.e. reduced time spent
  travelling, waiting for and
  consulting the physician and/or
  pharmacist)
	Other non-health benefits
	Value of information
	Value of reassurance
	Value of anxiety

	Process benefits Value of reduced travel time Value of reduced waiting time Value of seeing preferred NHS personnel

National Health Service staff costs would thus be reduced if more drugs were deregulated from prescription cost control.

Consumables are items which are used for or on behalf of each patient such as drugs, dressings, and disposable equipment. Consumables are replaced on a regular basis, hence unit costs are usually both appropriate and readily available. When switching drugs from prescription-only to OTC availability, the NHS does not pay the cost of the drug and therefore the drugs bill will be reduced.

Costs to patients, their families and their friends should be included when a societal approach is being adopted. Allowing pharmacists to supply more drugs through direct OTC sales offers potential savings to patients in the form of time and travel costs of visiting the physician (including savings in time spent in the waiting room and in the consultation itself). In terms of the actual monetary cost, all patients obtaining a drug directly from the pharmacist pay the retail price of the drug. However, if they obtain it on prescription, only a proportion of patients will pay the prescription charge. Thus, for some patients (e.g. those who are exempt from prescription charges and those for whom the cost of the recommended drug is greater than the prescription charge), the actual monetary cost of obtaining the drug will be higher when it is obtained from a pharmacist. Such patients may continue to obtain the drug from their physician, depending on the relative size of the time and travel costs.

The way pharmacists are paid should also be considered. Under the arrangements whereby the pharmaceutical service is currently administered, it is expected that a proportion of the pharmacist's income will be provided by commercial profit. There may therefore be an incentive for them to recommend more expensive drugs to patients, as well as larger quantity packs.

Money costs incurred should be valued at the actual amount. The opportunity cost of time depends on the alternative use of this resource. If this is paid employment then the value is proxied as the average wage rate; for unpaid labour the value is currently proxied at 54% of the average wage rate and for leisure time the value is taken as 43% of the average wage rate (Department of Transport, 1987).

Identifying and measuring benefits

Where drugs are made available OTC, there may be concerns that patients' health will deteriorate because pharmacists are not trained to diagnose. At present, pharmacists recommend treatments only for minor ailments. The adverse effects of such treatments, and hence any potential problems, are limited. Recent Government policy has reflected this, since drugs switched from prescription-only status to OTC availability have, in theory, been for the treatment of such minor ailments. This has already been discussed in the previous chapter. However, given that the pharmacists' undergraduate course is currently being extended to include more training in diagnosis and treatment for minor disease, future OTC drugs may include those for a wider variety of ailments. As long as the selection of drugs for deregulation is monitored closely, and the necessary education and information is provided, pharmacists will be able to advise and treat safely and effectively patients with a wider range of ailments. The health effects are therefore assumed to be negligible.

In terms of non-health benefits, there may be changes in information levels, reassurance levels, and anxiety levels (with patients receiving more or less of each of these attributes from their pharmacist compared to their doctor). Evidence from elsewhere suggests that such attributes are important to individuals in the provision of healthcare (Gerard *et al.*, 1992; Mooney and Lange, 1993; Mooney, 1994; Ryan, 1995; Donaldson *et al.*, 1995; Vick and Scott, 1998). In terms of process attributes, there is likely to be value to patients in terms of reductions in travel and waiting time, as well as a change in the staff that are involved in providing the drug. Again, this is supported by evidence from elsewhere (Propper, 1990; 1995; Ryan, 1995; Bryan *et al.*, 1998; Ryan, 1999).

Having identified benefits, attempts must be made to value them. The Quality Adjusted Life Year (QALY) paradigm dominated benefit assessment exercises throughout the 1980s (Williams, 1985; EuroQol, 1990; Kind *et al.*, 1994). This approach values improvements in health outcomes. Attempts to go beyond health outcomes, and take account of non-health outcomes and process attributes, led to the development and application of willingness to pay (WTP) and conjoint analysis (CA) in health economics. Given the nature of the potential benefits from switching drugs from prescription-only to OTC availability, the QALY paradigm is not likely to be sensitive to considering such benefits. Given this, the application of WTP and CA to this context is developed in this chapter.

Willingness to pay

According to the economic instrument of willingness to pay, the benefits to individuals from consuming a good are measured by their maximum willingness to pay (WTP) for that good. The technique of WTP is based on the premise that the maximum amount of money an individual is willing to pay for a commodity is an indicator of the utility or satisfaction to her/him of that commodity. It also has the advantage that individuals should consider all factors that are important to them in the provision of a good or service when considering their maximum WTP. Hence, they take account of health outcomes, non-health outcomes and process attributes. Using the economic instrument of willingness to pay, a demand schedule can be drawn, as shown in Figure 4.1 for the case of drugs. The demand schedule slopes downwards from left to right on the assumption that, as the cost per item falls, more consumers become willing to bear the cost, and the quantity of drugs demanded increases. (For evidence that the demand schedule for drugs is downward sloping see Ryan and Birch, 1991.) At a cost Pp per item, demand is Qp. Total WTP for Qp is represented by the area under the demand curve, ABQp0, and total costs by the area PpBQp0. The net benefit from consuming the drug is equal to the difference between what the individual is willing to pay and what they actually have to pay. This is represented by the difference between ABQp0 and PpBQp0 i.e. ABPp. This area is known as consumers'

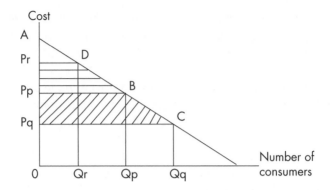

Figure 4.1 Demand schedule and consumer surplus for drugs. (Modified with permission from Ryan and Bond, 1996.)

surplus and can be simply defined as the difference between total WTP and total costs.

If the cost per item falls to Pq, demand increases to Qq, total WTP is then ACQq0, and total cost PqCQq0 and net benefits are ACPq. The gain in net benefits from the reduction in price is shown by the shaded area PpBCPq. Similarly, if cost per item increases to Pr, demand falls to Qr, total WTP is then ADQr0, total cost PrDQr0 and net benefits are ADPr. The loss in net benefits from the increase in cost is shown by the shaded area PrDBPp.

Figure 4.2 shows how these concepts can be used to estimate the benefits from switching drugs from prescription-only to OTC

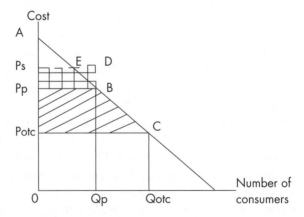

Figure 4.2 Estimating the benefits from switching drugs from prescription-only to over-the-counter availability

availability. The system of NHS charges complicates matters. The effect of these charges may be to subsidise or inflate the cost of drugs to patients. Here we assume that drugs are subsidised, since this is the case for many of the drugs switched to date.

In Figure 4.2, Pp is the cost to the patient of the drug on prescription, comprising the prescription charge plus time and travel costs. Ps is the cost to society of the drug on prescription, incorporating its cost to the Government (ingredient cost, dispensing fees paid to pharmacists and the value of general practitioners' time used), plus time and travel costs to patients. This does not include the prescription charge as this is a transfer payment (transferred from the patient to the Government). To include it would involve double counting. Our assumption that drugs are being subsidised means that Pp is less than Ps. When the drug is available only on prescription, the quantity dispensed is Qp and total benefits are ABQp0. Although the total cost to consumers is PpBQp0, the total cost to society is greater, at PsDQp0. So the net benefit to society is ABQp0 minus PsDQp0, or AEPs minus BDE.

Removing the restriction on OTC sales means that the drug can be obtained directly from the pharmacy at a cost of Potc (the product's retail price, plus time and travel costs to consumers of obtaining it from the pharmacy). We assume in Figure 4.2 that Potc is less than Pp. At the lower cost, demand increases to Qotc. This demand includes patients who would previously have obtained a prescription but now substitute an OTC purchase of the same product, as well as 'new' consumers who would not previously have obtained this product (or would have obtained a different product either on prescription or OTC). Total benefits to society after the switch are ACQotc0, and total costs are PotcCQotc0, so the net benefit is ACPotc.

The gain to society as a result of OTC availability can now be seen by comparing the net benefits before and after the policy change. This is shown by the shaded area PsDBCPotc. Strictly, this assumes that all individuals face the same time and money costs; thus if one patient finds it advantageous to obtain the drug OTC rather than on prescription, all will do so. In reality, of course, people face different costs, and only if Potc is less than Pp for the individual will it be worthwhile for them to 'switch'.

Conjoint analysis

Conjoint analysis can be used to estimate the value of different attributes in the provision of a good or service, as well as how individuals trade these attributes, and WTP for individual attributes if cost is included as an attribute. Whilst the technique is well established in the market research literature, and is widely used in transport economics and environmental economics (Ryan, 1995), it is only just beginning to be used in health economics (Propper, 1990; 1995; Ryan, 1995; Ryan and Hughes, 1997; van der Pol and Cairns, 1997; Bryan *et al.*, 1998; Ryan *et al.*, 1998; Vick and Scott, 1998; Ryan, 1999). Its increased use in health economics can be partly explained by the desire for a technique that can take account of more than health outcomes. Using CA, preferences may be elicited using ranking, rating or discrete choice exercises. The approach currently favoured by economists is the discrete choice approach, partly because it incorporates the notion of sacrifice. Here the individual is asked to make numerous choices between two options, A and B, which may vary with regard to health attributes, non-health attributes and process attributes, or any combination of these. An example of a discrete choice question used to evaluate alternative systems for repeat prescribing (Bond *et al.*, 1997) is provided in Figure 4.3. Regression techniques are used to analyse the responses. From this regression equation it is possible to establish: (i) the relative importance of individual attributes in the provision of a product or service; (ii) the trade-offs that individuals are willing to make between these attributes; and (iii) WTP for these attributes if cost is included as an attribute.

Attributes	System A	System B
Convenience of ordering and collecting your medicines	You attend the surgery and visit the pharmacy	You visit the pharmacy only
Cost of ordering and collecting your repeat prescriptions	£2.00 per month	£1.00 per month
Quality of advice received when collecting your repeat medicines	No advice	Spoken directions

	Prefer System A	Prefer System B
Which system do you prefer?	☐	☐

Figure 4.3   Example of discrete choice question in a conjoint analysis exercise

Empirical evidence

Although there has been a general increase in the availability of OTC drugs supplied by pharmacists in the UK, very little attention has been given to the economic implications of these policies, although issues raised when debating extending the role of pharmacists have been described (Ryan and Bond, 1994; Fryklof, 1994; Axon, 1994; Ahlgrimm, 1994; Anderson, 1994; Takemasa, 1994; Gerbrands, 1994). To date there have been no randomised controlled trials (RCTs) looking at the costs and benefits of reclassifying drugs.

Economic demand theory has been applied to attempt to estimate the benefits from switching drugs from prescription-only availability to being available OTC (Temin, 1983; Ryan and Yule, 1990; Ryan and Yule, 1992). Temin (1983) applied the theory to look at the benefits of switching 0.5% topical hydrocortisone in the US in 1979. His study was conducted three years after the drug was switched. He noted that prescription sales did not fall when the drug became available OTC, and that the resulting demand could therefore be seen as a net expansion of the market for the drug. The added sales to this 'new market' were estimated to be 11.79 million units in 1980, 24.12 million units in 1981 and 28 million units in 1982. The average price of these units was estimated by dividing the total value of the OTC sales by the number of sales. This gave an average price of $3.57 in 1980, $2.91 in 1981 and $2.80 in 1982. Within the US, the cost of the drug on prescription is made up of the price of the drug, the cost of the doctor visit needed to get the prescription, and the value of the consumer's time to go to the doctor. Temin assumed that the first of these is the same on prescription and OTC. The doctor's fee was estimated to be $30 and the value of consumer's time $10, giving a cost difference before and after the switch of $40. Assuming a linear demand function, consumer surplus was estimated to be $236 million for 1980 (1/2 × $40 × 11.79), $482 million for 1981 (1/2 × $40 × 24.12) and $560 million for 1982 (1/2 × $40 × 28).

Ryan and Yule (1990) applied the economic theory of consumer surplus to assess the benefits of switching two drugs from prescription-only to OTC availability in the UK – loperamide and 1% topical hydrocortisone. To apply the theory to these drugs the following information was needed: costs (time and money) to consumers of obtaining drugs on prescription and OTC; the cost of each drug to society; the demand for each drug before and after the switch; and the degree of substitution of OTC sales for prescriptions.

Time costs of obtaining drugs were estimated using data on average distances travelled to the general practitioner's surgery and pharmacy by different modes of transport (Ritchie *et al.*, 1981). It was assumed that people walk on average three miles per hour and that private and public transport travels at 20 miles per hour. Average waiting time in the general practitioner's surgery was taken to be 13.6 minutes (OPCS, 1982), and the average length of a general practitioner consultation to be five minutes (Westcott, 1977; Raynes and Cairns, 1980). Waiting and consultation times at the pharmacy were assumed to be negligible. The UK Department of Transport's value of leisure time, 153.2 p per hour (Department of Transport, 1987), was used to value individuals' time. An approximate value for general practitioners' time was derived by dividing their average recommended earnings by their average hours of work.

Net ingredient costs and retail prices of drugs were obtained from the Chemist and Druggist Price List and the Monthly Index of Medical Specialities (MIMS), and pharmacists' fees were calculated according to the Drug Tariff. It was assumed that individuals purchased the largest OTC packs and that the same pack sizes would have been obtained on prescription. To determine average travelling expenses, bus fares were valued at 2p per minute and, for private transport, a cost of 30p per mile was employed.

Data on OTC sales of loperamide and 1% topical hydrocortisone were obtained from their manufacturers. To estimate the extent to which these sales substituted for NHS prescriptions, levels of prescribing before and after the policy changes were compared. Prescribing data were supplied by the Department of Health (Statistics and Research Division).

Information was collected on the number of prescriptions for loperamide and 1% topical hydrocortisone from 1980 to 1987. When loperamide became available OTC in 1983, prescribing fell in relation to its previous trend, suggesting that OTC sales were substituted for prescriptions. Extrapolating the growth rate from 1980–83 (17% per year), it would have been expected that 1.025 million prescriptions would have been dispensed in 1985, 1.200 million in 1986 and 1.403 million in 1987. Comparing this with actual prescribing implies that prescription numbers were reduced by 0.280 million in 1985, 0.401 million in 1986 and 0.549 million in 1987. Given total OTC sales of 1.361 million packs in 1985, 1.350 million in 1986 and 1.959 million in 1987, estimated numbers of 'new' customers were 1.081 million, 0.949 million and 1.410 million, respectively.

There was no clear change in the number of prescriptions for topical hydrocortisone in 1987 following the introduction of an OTC substitute. This may reflect the fact that only a short period had elapsed since the policy change, though Temin (1983) similarly found no effect on prescribing when OTC sales of topical hydrocortisone were introduced in the US. OTC sales of this drug, 1.100 million packs in 1987, were viewed as a 'new' market.

Costs of obtaining loperamide and 1% topical hydrocortisone on prescription and OTC are shown in Table 4.2. On this basis, the benefits from over-the-counter availability of loperamide were £2.8 million in 1985, £2.9 million in 1986 and £4.2 million in 1987 (all at 1987 prices). The corresponding benefits for 1% topical hydrocortisone were £2.0 million in 1987.

Temin (1983) attempted to quantify the costs from the OTC availability of topical hydrocortisone. He argued that adverse drug reactions would be limited, since anyone experiencing them would be immediately aware and would stop using the cream. This would, however, lead to a cost in terms of the value of unused cream. Costs may also be incurred if the consumer sees a doctor to diagnose any drug reactions. Given that there are no data in this area, Temin argued that a conservative estimate was to deduct 10% of the benefit to allow for these costs. He argued that, given the topical nature of the drug, this adjustment was generous. Making this adjustment, the net benefits of switching topical hydrocortisone were estimated to be $212 million in 1980, $433 million in 1981 and $504 million in 1982.

Ryan and Yule (1990) did not estimate the costs from the wider availability of loperamide and hydrocortisone. They do note, however, that the side effects and adverse reactions from these drugs are usually held to be limited (Edwards and Stillman, 1987; Mehta, 1999), though this has been disputed (Winfield and Mackintosh, 1987). Applying the assumption that Temin made that the costs incurred are 10% of the benefits, the net benefits from the wider availability of loperamide are

Table 4.2 Costs of obtaining loperamide and 1% topical hydrocortisone on prescription and over-the-counter (£) (1987 prices)

		Prescription charge	P_p	Retail price	P_{otc}	P_s
Loperamide	1985	2.15	5.77	1.55	2.47	6.24
Loperamide	1986	2.20	5.91	1.89	2.81	6.28
Loperamide	1987	2.40	6.02	1.97	2.89	6.61
Topical hydrocortisone	1987	2.40	6.02	1.49	2.41	6.18

estimated to be £3.15 million in 1985, £3.3 million in 1986 and £5 million in 1987. The corresponding benefit for 1% topical hydrocortisone is £2 million in 1987, £1.9 million in 1988 and £2 million in 1989.

Discussion and conclusion

Recent years have seen a relaxing of the legislation restricting certain drugs to prescription-only availability. This chapter has considered some of the issues raised in looking at the costs and benefits of this policy. Relaxing the legislation on the availability of drugs directly from the pharmacist will lead to savings in patient time and travel costs. Given the system of NHS charges, the effect on the money price the patient pays for the drug is unclear. Given that there is no system in operation other than professional responsibility or market pressures that may curb the incentive for pharmacists to provide more drugs of a higher cost, patients may pay a higher monetary cost under a system of prescribing pharmacists. Such a system would, however, result in savings in GP time and dispensing costs to the Government. There are concerns that the pharmacist is not currently trained to advise on treatment other than for minor, self-limiting conditions. However, given the recent extensions to pharmacists' undergraduate training, there may be a role in the future for OTC drugs to be extended to include those for a wider variety of ailments. Such deregulation should continue to be closely monitored.

As some of the drugs proposed for deregulation might have the capacity to be recommended inappropriately, the professional bodies have already expressed their concerns and are monitoring the situation closely (Scottish Department Executive, 1992). There have been reports criticising the advice provided by community pharmacists in response to symptoms, such as the management of childhood diarrhoea (Goodburn *et al.*, 1991), although the *agent provocateur* methodology used in this particular study has been strongly criticised because of the lack of realism when a covert researcher pays the role of a patient seeking advice. However, in Australia, where salbutamol (albuterol) inhalers have been available from pharmacies since 1985 (although their deregulation in the UK and US was abandoned because of lack of medical support), there is some evidence of inadequate treatment for patients obtaining their inhalers from pharmacies (Gibson *et al.*, 1993). The recommendations for the treatment of asthma have recently changed in Australia, the UK, the US and elsewhere. Thus, many patients who previously self-medicated on bronchodilators would ideally be treated with inhaled steroids, which are available only on medical prescription.

In the light of the availability of bronchodilators OTC, when the recommendations for treatment were changed, pharmacists should have been provided with clear guidelines specifying exclusions to treatment, length of treatment and for when to refer patients to general practitioners. This sort of model has already been successfully piloted for the OTC treatment of dyspepsia. Clinical pharmacy protocols have been developed by a group of pharmacists, general practitioners, a pharmacologist and a gastroenterologist; these protocols include the re-classified H_2-blockers as one possible treatment (Bond *et al.*, 1993). This is described in detail in Chapter 3.

It was shown that very little empirical work has addressed these issues. Given the absence of any detailed modelling of the demand for individual drugs, what work is available has made use of readily available data, and attempted to predict the change in demand following the policy change by comparing levels of prescribing before and after the policy change. What is clearly needed to apply the theory of consumer surplus in the future is developed models of demand for individual drugs. In the absence of actual data sets to do this modelling, a way forward is to use what economists call stated preference data sets. Here, rather than use actual market data, as was used in the studies by Temin and Ryan and Yule, individuals are asked to state their preferences within a hypothetical setting.

Within the context of WTP studies individuals would be asked a hypothetical question concerning their maximum WTP for a drug for which a prescription was obtained initially from the doctor and dispensed by the pharmacist, and their WTP for a drug obtained directly from the pharmacist. Whilst no studies to date have applied the WTP instrument to look at the benefits of switching drugs from prescription only to OTC availability, a number of such studies have applied the instrument to assessing the value of different drug regimens (Reardon and Pathak, 1990; Johannesson and Jonsson, 1991; Johannesson and Fagerberg, 1992; Johannesson *et al.*, 1993; O'Brien *et al.*, 1995; O'Brien *et al.*, 1998). Within the area of pharmacy, Gore and Madhavan (1994) used WTP to look at consumer preferences for pharmacist counselling for non-prescription medicines, Einarson *et al.* (1988) to look at the value of establishing a serum cholesterol monitoring service in a community pharmacy and Silcock *et al.* (1999) to look at consumer preference for advice on smoking cessation (see Chapter 8).

Using the discrete choice CA approach, individuals would be presented with numerous discrete choices which varied with respect to the attributes that differ between obtaining the prescription from the doctor or the drug directly from the pharmacist. Based on what has been said in this paper, these include: who authorises the drug (doctor or pharmacist); travel time; waiting time and money costs. An example of a discrete choice question is presented in Figure 4.4. The individual would be presented with numerous choices and, for each, asked which system they preferred. From the responses it would be possible to estimate the relative importance of the different attributes, how individuals trade between these attributes, and WTP for the different systems.

To date no studies have taken place using CA to look at the benefits of reclassifying drugs. However, Bond *et al.* (1997) used the technique within a RCT to look at patient preferences concerning the introduction of a new repeat prescribing system whereby the community pharmacist monitored and controlled repeat prescribing. (For an example of a discrete choice question from this study see Figure 4.3.) This study found that respondents in the intervention group of the trial preferred to collect their prescription directly from the pharmacist, and that they were willing to pay £1.50 extra for this (see Chapter 5).

An important assumption of demand theory (which underlies both WTP and CA) is that individuals have reasonably good information about the advantages and disadvantages of consuming the product.

Attributes	System A	System B
Drug system	Doctor prescribes and pharmacist dispenses	Available directly from the pharmacist
Travel time	15 minutes	5 minutes
Waiting time	15 minutes	3 minutes
Consultation time	10 minutes	2 minutes
Cost of drug	£5.00	£2.50

	Prefer System A	Prefer System B
Which system do you prefer?	☐	☐

Figure 4.4 Example of discrete choice question in a conjoint analysis exercise looking at the benefits of extending the role of the pharmacist

Drugs most likely to satisfy these requirements will be those for relatively minor ailments, where consumers are competent to diagnose the complaint and monitor the effects of treatment. Whilst this is plausible for drugs for minor ailments, it would be less so for drugs for serious ailments or drugs with complex pharmacological effects.

In conclusion, increasing the role of pharmacists so that they can directly supply more drugs is likely to save money for both the NHS and some patients. A reassessment of the legal status of drugs and subsequent OTC switch of drugs used to treat minor self-limiting illnesses is therefore encouraged. However, there may be drawbacks associated with this system should deregulation extend beyond the range of drugs that are safe and that selectively treat minor self-limiting symptomatic conditions.

Acknowledgements

Financial support from the Medical Research Council and Chief Scientist Office of the Scottish Home and Health Department and the University of Aberdeen are acknowledged. The opinions expressed are those of the author.

References

Ahlgrimm E D (1994). Dispensing doctors and prescribing pharmacists, the German situation. *J Soc Admin Pharm* 11: 112–15.

Anderson L J (1994). Dispensing doctors and prescribing pharmacists in the USA. *J Soc Admin Pharm* 11: 116–20.

Axon S R (1994). Dispensing doctors – an international perspective. *J Soc Admin Pharm* 11: 106–11.

Bond C M, Winfield A (1993). Pharmacists' protocols. *Report to the Scottish Office Home and Health Department*. Department of General Practice, University of Aberdeen.

Bond C, Matheson C, Jones J, *et al.* (1997). *Repeat prescribing study*. Final Report submitted to Scottish Office, Project No 4–024.

Bryan S, Buxton M, Sheldon R, *et al.* (1998). Magnetic resonance imaging for the investigation of knee injuries: an investigation of preference. *Health Econ* 7: 595–604.

Department of Transport (1987). *Value for journey time savings and accident prevention*. London: Department of Transport.

Donaldson C, Shackley P (1997). Economic evaluation. In: Detels R, Holland W, McEwan J, *et al.*, eds. *Oxford Textbook of Public Health*, 3rd edn. Oxford: Oxford University Press.

Donaldson C, Shackley P, Abdalla M, *et al.* (1995). Willingness to pay for antenatal carrier screening for cystic fibrosis. *Health Econ* 4: 439–52.

Edwards C, Stillman P (1987). The use of topical hydrocortisone. *Pharm J* 238: 169–74.

Einarson T R, Bootman J L, McGhan W F, et al. (1988). Establishment and evaluation of a serum cholesterol monitoring service in a community pharmacy. *Drug Intell Clin Pharm* 22: 45–8.

EuroQol (1990). EuroQol – a new facility for the measurement of health-related quality of life. *Health Policy* 16: 199–208.

Fryklof L E (1994). Dispensing Doctors and Prescribing Pharmacists – Where is the Borderline? *J Soc Admin Pharm* 11: 105.

Gerard K, Turnbull D, Lange M, et al. (1992). Economic evaluation of mammography screening: Information, reassurance and anxiety. *Health Economics Research Unit Discussion Paper* No. 01/92, Aberdeen: University of Aberdeen.

Gibson P, Henry D, Francis L, et al. (1993). Association between availability of non-prescription β_2-agonist inhalers and undertreatment of asthma. *BMJ* 306: 1514–18.

Goodburn E, Mattosinho S, Mongi P, et al. (1991). Management of childhood diarrhoea by pharmacists and parents: is Britain lagging behind the Third World? *BMJ* 302: 440–43.

Gore P R, Madhavan S (1994). Consumers' preferences and willingness to pay for pharmacist counselling for non-prescription medicines. *J Clin Pharm Ther* 19: 17–25.

Johannesson M, Fagerberg B (1992). A health economic comparison of diet and drug treatment in obese men with mid hypertension. *J Hypertens* 10: 1063–70.

Johannesson M, Jonsson B, Borgquist L (1991). Willingness to pay for antihypertensive therapy – results of a Swedish pilot study. *Journal of Health Economics* 10: 461–74.

Johannesson M, Johansson P-O, Kristrom B, et al. (1993). Willingness to pay for antihypertensive therapy – further results. *Journal of Health Economics* 12: 95–108.

Kind P, Dolan P, Gudex C, et al. (1994). Practical and methodological issues in the development of the EuroQol: the York experience. *Advances in Medical Sociology* 5: 219–53.

Mehta D K, ed. (1999). *British National Formulary* 38. London: British Medical Association and Royal Pharmaceutical Society of Great Britain.

Mooney G (1994). What else do we want from our health services? *Soc Sci Med* 39: 151–54.

Mooney G, Lange M (1993). Ante-natal screening: What constitutes benefit? *Soc Sci Med* 37: 873–78.

O'Brien B, Novosel S, Torrance G, et al. (1995). Assessing the economic value of a new antidepressant. *PharmacoEconomics* 8: 34–45.

O'Brien B, Goeree R, Gafni A, et al. (1998). Assessing the value of a new pharmaceutical: a feasibility study of contingent valuation in managed care. *Med Care* 36: 370–84.

Office of Population Censuses and Surveys (1982). London: HMSO.

Propper C (1990). Contingent valuation of time spent on NHS waiting lists. *Economic Journal* 100: 193–99.

Propper C (1995). The disutility of time spent on the United Kingdom's National Health Service waiting lists. *Journal of Human Resources* 30: 677–700.

Ratcliffe J, Ryan M, Tucker J (1996). The costs of alternative types of routine antenatal care for low risk women: shared care vs care by general practitioners and community midwives. *Journal of Health Services Research and Policy* 1: 135–40.

Raynes N V, Cairns V (1980). Factors contributing to the length of the general practice consultation. *J R Coll Gen Pract* 30: 496.

Reardon G, Pathalk D S (1990). Segmenting the antihistamine market: an investigation of consumer preferences. *Journal of Health Care and Marketing* 10: 23–33.

Ritchie J, Jacoby A, Bone M (1981). *Access to primary care* London: HMSO.

Ryan M (1995). *Economics and the patient's utility function: an application to Assisted Reproductive Techniques.* PhD Thesis, University of Aberdeen, Aberdeen.

Ryan M (1999). Using conjoint analysis to take account of patient preferences and go beyond health outcomes: an application to in vitro fertilisation. *Soc Sci Med* 48: 535–46.

Ryan M, Birch S (1991). Charging for health care: evidence on the utilisation of NHS prescribed drugs. *Soc Sci Med* 33: 681–87.

Ryan M, Bond C (1994). Dispensing physicians and prescribing pharmacists: economic considerations for the UK. *PharmacoEconomics* 5: 8–17.

Ryan M, Bond C M (1996). Using the economic theory of consumer surplus to estimate the benefits of dispensing doctors and prescribing pharmacists. *J Soc Admin Pharm* 13(4): 178–87.

Ryan M, Hughes J (1997). Using conjoint analysis to assess women's preferences for miscarriage management. *Health Econ* 6: 261–73.

Ryan M, Yule B (1990). Switching drugs from prescription-only to over-the-counter availability: economic benefits in the United Kingdom. *Health Policy* 16: 233–39.

Ryan M, Yule B (1992). Benefits from switching drugs from prescription-only to over-the-counter availability: the UK experience. In: Huttin C, Bosanquet N, eds. *The prescription drug market: international perspectives and challenges for the future.* Holland: North Holland.

Ryan M, McIntosh E, Shackley P (1998). Using conjoint analysis to assess consumer preferences in primary care: an application to the patient health card. *Health Expectations* 1: 117–29.

Scottish Department Executive (1992). Report on council meeting of the Royal Pharmaceutical Society. *Pharm J* 248: 219.

Sinclair H K, Bond C M, Silcock J, *et al.* (1999). The cost effectiveness of intensive pharmaceutical intervention in assisting people to stop smoking. *Int J Phar Pract* 7: 107–12.

Takemasa F (1994). The contrasting philosophies of Eastern and Western Pharmacy: Meeting of the ways. *J Soc Adm Pharm* 11: 121–26.

Temin P (1983). Costs and benefits of switching drugs from Rx to OTC. *Journal of Health Economics* 2: 187–205.

van der Pol M, Cairns J (1998). Establishing patient preferences for blood transfusion support: an application of conjoint analysis. *Journal Health Services Research and Policy* 3: 70–6.

Vick S, Scott A (1998). Agency in health care: examining patients' preferences for attributes of the doctor-patient relationship. *Journal of Health Economics* 17: 587–606.

Westcott R (1977). The length of the consultation in general practice. *J R Coll Gen Pract* 27: 552.

Williams A (1985). Economics of coronary artery bypass grafting. *BMJ* 291: 326–29.

Winfield A J, Mackintosh J M (1987). An evaluation of community pharmacists' knowledge of OTC hydrocortisone. *British Journal of Pharmaceutical Practice*, 9: 434–36, 444.

5

Prescribing

Christine Bond

General practice prescribing

Background

General practice prescribing accounts for over 10% of the national UK NHS budget and 60% of spending in primary care. It has been criticised by both academic and national bodies (National Audit Office, 1994; National Audit Office, 1993). In Scotland prescribing-related issues are identified as being central to improved primary care in the long-term context of healthcare changes (Scottish Office, 1993). Repeat prescribing accounts for approximately 75% of all general practice prescribed items and 80% of all costs on primary care medicines (Harris and Dajda, 1996). It is estimated that repeat prescribing affects 20% of all patients receiving a prescription. Many patients are on polypharmacy regimens. Current practice for generating repeat prescriptions, either computer or receptionist written, are generally acknowledged to provide inadequate control, resulting in overprescribing, stockpiling of drugs and infrequent review of therapy (National Audit Office, 1993), which may lead to failure to identify issues such as drug interactions, adverse drug reactions, poor compliance and inappropriate treatment.

A repeat prescription, in contrast to an acute prescription, has been defined as 'a prescription for a chronic or recurrent condition issued without a clinical review'. In some contexts it is also taken to designate those prescriptions issued by computer from a repeat prescribing programme (Harris and Dajda, 1996; Zermansky, 1996). Neither of these is likely to include face-to-face consultation with the doctor or clinical review of notes. Increasingly, this procedure is carried out by practice administration staff, with a typical mechanism being that when a patient is stabilised on a medication, as determined by the general practitioner, they are added to the repeat prescribing register for the practice. When further supplies of the medication are required, the patient contacts the surgery, either by letter, a phone call or a personal visit, and requests the items needed for continuation of therapy. The receptionist is then responsible for generating a further prescription, most often, but not necessarily, through the general practice computer system. Prescriptions produced in this way should be attached to the patients' notes before presenting to the general practitioner for signature. In practice, because of the volume of such prescriptions, a pile of 'repeats' is signed at 'coffee time' by each general practitioner in the practice on a rota basis, and clinical control is minimal. The detailed lack of controls have been listed recently (Zermansky, 1996). Problems may arise because the general practitioner signing the prescription is often not familiar with the patient and does not have the time to check the notes. Such lack of controls has given rise to a range of anecdotes of prescriptions being signed for items such as a 'pound of mince'. *The Pharmaceutical Journal* regularly reports on such nonsensical prescriptions (Anonymous, 1992a; Anonymous, 1992b), which computerisation has not eliminated (Anonymous, 1992c). Another problem with this system is that general practitioners take it in turns for their personalised ciphered prescription forms to be used for the repeat prescribing shift. Thus, because of the high proportion of items which are repeats, computerised feedback of prescribing statistics (e.g. Prescribing Analysis and Costs (PACT) in England and Wales and Scottish Prescribing Analysis (SPA) in Scotland) cannot be more than practice specific.

Another problem resulting from current mechanisms is that, because of the workload for general practice staff, the duration of the medication supply for an individual patient on a single prescription form is steadily increasing. This may also be partly a function of the steady increase in the prescription levy, and the inclination of some general practitioners to 'take the law into their own hands' and provide more drugs at a time, thus reducing the number of levies collected. Thus, whereas at one time a month's supply per prescription form would be the norm, three-monthly supplies are often recorded. This is one of the causes of the stockpiling and wastage of medicines. There are also short-term implications for the remuneration of pharmacists, whose income is largely dependent on prescription volume (see Note 1, p. 112). Thus, an ideal system would need to be able to introduce monthly clinical controls into the process without an undue increase in general practitioner workload.

In the Irish Republic a scheme to achieve this was introduced in 1996. For suitable patients, general practitioners issue a triplicate copy of the prescription which is stored in the community pharmacy and dispensed in three instalments. The pharmacist is remunerated for handling each instalment, regardless of whether an item is dispensed; thus, if it is identified that the patient does not need further supplies, the pharmacist can refuse to dispense the next instalment (Irish Pharmaceutical Contractors Committee, 1996).

An ideal system might be one in which a general practitioner would first stabilise a patient for a chronic medication regimen, then decide, on the basis of clinical judgement only, when s/he would like to review that regimen. This might depend on a range of factors, such as: the need for monitoring for drug side effects (e.g. haematology); monitoring for treatment efficacy; the nature of the illness; and the stability of the patient's condition. There are also patient factors to consider, such as personality, mental ability and lay support. Having assessed these factors, the general practitioner should be able to write, for example, a 12-month prescription, with directions to be dispensed monthly. Interim clinical controls could then be delivered at each dispensing by the community pharmacist, who could check on drug efficacy, side effects and the need for continued treatment; this latter point could allow support for compliance issues and address drug wastage. Ideally, the community pharmacist could also consider a systematic review of all the patient's medication needs. An alternative could be for a pharmacist based within the general practice setting to review a patient's medication in the practice.

At the moment both of these mechanisms are in use in various parts of the UK to a greater or lesser extent. It may be that in future a range of models will be in place, tailored to the needs of the patient.

Control of repeat prescribing as suggested here is another example of the increased involvement of the community pharmacist in primary healthcare, interfacing both with the general practitioner and directly with the general public (Department of Health, 1987; Bond *et al.*, 1995; Bond *et al.*, 2000). A survey of Grampian general practitioners' attitudes towards various extended roles which have been proposed for the community pharmacist (Bond *et al.*, 1995) demonstrated that only a third of respondents were not in favour of repeat prescribing by the pharmacist following agreed protocols. In a subsequent workshop there was overwhelming consensus to assess the pharmaceutical control of repeat prescribing and the use of instalment dispensing was identified as a mechanism by which this could be implemented within the current legislation.

The research issues

The introduction of the Irish system described above could be criticised because it represented a significant change from previous practice yet it had not been tested or evaluated. One of the possible reasons for the lack of feasibility pilot projects could be a result of the problems in researching an area which is clearly controlled by statute and regulation.

In such circumstances, any feasibility study can only mimic the long-term implementation proposed. Thus in repeat prescribing, greater involvement of the community pharmacist may require multiple prescription forms to be produced and signed individually by the general practitioner; a tiresome task. In Scotland, a modification of the instalment dispensing process (see Note 2, p. 113) could also be used. This mechanism is somewhat similar to the repeat mechanism for private prescriptions. A total prescribed quantity can be ordered, with specified amounts to be dispensed at monthly intervals. The original intent of the 'instalment' procedure was to allow drug misusers on substitute medication to receive their dispensed supplies on a daily basis. However, the regulations are such that it may be used more generally.

Another problem when carrying out research in this area is its effect on change in prescription form volume, and the implications this has for community pharmacists' remuneration. Issues in relation to these topics have been discussed elsewhere (Bond *et al.*, 1997).

Assuming that a feasibility study can be established in spite of the above constraints, what are the research questions? In such a situation there are four interested 'stakeholders', namely the general practitioner, the pharmacist, the patient and the NHS. The sort of things that need to be evaluated are:

For the general practitioner:

- Will the pharmacist follow an agreed protocol to check appropriateness of supply at each dispensing?
- Will there be a conflict of interest for the pharmacist?
- Will there be any effect on prescribing costs?
- What are the workload implications for general practitioner and practice staff?

For the pharmacist:

- What will be the effect on workload?
- What will be the effect on remuneration?
- What are the advantages to the pharmacist?

For the patient:

- Do they understand the new scheme?
- Do they like the new scheme?
- Is the scheme convenient?

And for the NHS:

- Are there any changes in drug costs?
- Is there an increased identification of adverse drug reactions which could lead to reduced hospital admissions?
- What is the overall cost benefit ratio?

The methods

The research issues identified above include a combination of opinion, satisfaction, workload, outcome and health economic issues.

Opinion is often addressed through the use of a standard survey form which would ask for experiences of the new system and satisfaction with it. Because some of this sort of information may be highly biased due to one or two high impact events, it is important to validate key issues wherever possible by qualitative data extraction using either existing documents, such as patient records, or specifically designed prospective record cards.

However, patient opinion/satisfaction is not ideally evaluated in this way. Patient satisfaction, with whatever aspect of healthcare, is notoriously difficult to measure because of: patients' loyalty to practitioners; fear of retaliation if they indicate dissatisfaction; low expectations; lack of understanding of potential service. Thus, subtler techniques have to be employed to address these issues. One such example of this, developed for use in healthcare evaluation, is conjoint analysis. This technique, originally used in market research of non-healthcare services such as public transport, invites respondents repeatedly to state a preference for one service against another. Examples of two such comparisons are explained in Chapter 4.

Because of the complexity of the questions it is difficult for the patient to pick the 'correct' answer, and so a truer indication of the patient's preferences can be obtained. In a feasibility study such as the evaluation of a new service which had been experienced by the respondents, supporting factual information such as travel costs and times should also be collected and included in the conjoint analysis.

Changes in workload have to be based on more than opinion and should include 'before' and 'after' monitoring of the actual time taken to deliver the service. In a large study, pragmatism may dictate that self-timing using an agreed procedure and standardised data collection forms will suffice. Such self-reporting can be validated against objective random checks by the researcher, probably focusing on those practitioners with the greatest involvement. It is important, however, that 'work study' measurement should be carried out over a sufficient period of time to minimise variations due to time of day, time of the week, or seasonal factors.

Outcome measures vary between studies. In a study of repeat prescribing, it is important to look at both process and clinical outcomes. Thus, it would be ideal to monitor, for example, the number of compliance issues or adverse drug reaction/drug interactions which the individual community pharmacist identified. This can be done by a pharmacy-completed patient record card, which has the dual purpose of being part of the pharmaceutical care of the patient, as well as being a research record. Similar information from the general practitioners' perspectives can be collected from the patients' medical records.

Finally, health economic measures need collection of all the appropriate information. In this study, the workload factors, clinical outcomes, drug cost avoidance and patient direct and indirect costs would all contribute to health economic assessment of the intervention.

Any study involving patients must be submitted to a local ethics committee for approval. This is particularly the case if patients will be sent a questionnaire, or have their method of medication supply changed, or their medical records selected and searched. Thus, studies of new methods of repeat prescribing would almost certainly need to be passed by ethical committees. This includes not just the details of the study design, but often requires sample questionnaires, patient information sheets and patient consent forms. This will become increasingly important when the Caldicott Report (Department of Health, 1999) on patient confidentiality is implemented. Ways are currently being sought to promote patients' rights to privacy without preventing any patient-related research being undertaken.

Finally, what sort of study design would be best to evaluate a new method of repeat prescribing? Because so many of the outcomes could be affected by other factors, a randomised controlled design is the most suitable to try and eliminate confounders such as external circulars about reducing drug wastage, increasing compliance, identifying particular drug-related adverse reactions or side effects.

The study

In this section, we report on a study carried out in 1995 to evaluate a system in which community pharmacists monitored and controlled repeat prescribing. The points covered in the previous section should be illustrated by the study description.

Aims

The prime aim of the study was to assess the feasibility of community pharmacists controlling repeat prescribing by assessing the implications for patient, community pharmacist, general practitioner and the NHS.

Specific objectives were to evaluate: improvements to patient care with respect to the identification of drug interactions and drug-related adverse events; monitoring and improving patient compliance; benefits to the NHS with respect to reduced wastage of drugs, changes in non-elective hospital admission rates, possible changes in administrative costs; the wider implications for the patient, the NHS, community pharmacist, and general practitioner and practice manager.

Methods

Study design

This was a randomised controlled trial of a new service provided by community pharmacists to monitor and authorise the repeat dispensing of further supplies of medicines. The mechanism which was used to carry out the study within the current legislation was instalment dispensing. The study was discussed extensively with representatives of the Scottish Office, the Pharmacy Practice Division, the Joint Ethical Committee, the GP subcommittee of the Local Medical Committee and the Area Pharmaceutical Committee.

Recruitment of professionals

Every general practitioner in Grampian was invited to participate in the study in November 1994. Only those practices where every member of the practice was willing to participate were included in the study. Each interested practice was visited by a member of the project team to provide more details of the study. Practices were stratified by location, number of partners and current duration of repeat prescriptions and then randomly allocated to either the control or intervention group. The control group continued with their current method of issuing repeat prescriptions and the intervention group changed a sample of patients to the new system. Nineteen practices were recruited, nine intervention (36 general practitioners) and ten control (35 general practitioners).

All community pharmacists in Grampian (n = 121) were kept informed during general practitioner practice recruitment, and a list of the intervention group practices was circulated as soon as these had been identified. In rural locations, pharmacists were specifically asked if they would be willing to participate. Every community pharmacy which was likely to receive a 'study' prescription was visited before the study started.

Sixty-two community pharmacies across Grampian expected to receive prescriptions for patients recruited to the intervention group. Pharmacists in the catchment area of the intervention general practitioners were invited to attend one of four meetings at which the logistics and documentation of the study were presented and refined by consensus.

The intervention

Patients were provided with sufficient prescriptions to last until a review date, which was set by the general practitioner (for example, six months or 12 months) according to the patient's clinical need. For logistical reasons and to minimise cash flow implications for the community pharmacist, multiples of 'three-monthly' monthly instalment prescriptions were issued, kept by the community pharmacist and dispensed at monthly intervals. When the prescriptions were completed, the patient returned to the general practitioner for a medical review. The process was then repeated. Patients could take prescriptions to the pharmacy of their choice.

A protocol to assess patients for compliance, side effects, drug interactions and adverse events was agreed jointly by pharmacists and general practitioners. Information was recorded on specially designed summary cards retained by the pharmacist.

Patient recruitment

All patients currently on repeat medication were eligible for this study. They were included if they met the study inclusion criteria and were not excluded by the exclusion criteria. Patient recruitment took place between June 1995 and September 1995. Target recruitment was 250 patients for each practice. As patients requested their repeat medication, the first five patients were recruited daily. This was done over a ten-week period to spread and minimise workload for the practice staff and to ensure proper representation of the patient population on repeat medication. Practices in the control group recruited patients in the same way and 2380 patients were recruited before exclusion criteria applied. Exclusion criteria were applied at the point of data collection, to reduce the practice workload associated with patient recruitment.

Communication with professionals

All community pharmacists were contacted by telephone on at least two occasions throughout the 12-month study period to check on the progress of the study, identify and, where possible, resolve problems. Pharmacists were also visited at least once during the study. The purpose of this was again to identify and resolve any procedural problems, to check on the completion of the study documentation and to assess the numbers of study prescriptions held by each community pharmacist. Formal records were kept of all these telephone calls and visits and used to add in-depth information to the study evaluation. To inform and motivate professionals involved in the study, newsletters were circulated to community pharmacists and general practitioners three times throughout the study period.

Outcome measures

Process For the intervention patients, data were collected by community pharmacists at the point of dispensing on: suspected compliance problems; adverse reactions/drug interactions; other symptoms/problems. For a sample of 100 intervention patients from each practice (56% of total) and all control patients, general practice notes were searched for information on the number of general practice visits, compliance problems, adverse drug reactions, therapy changes, non-elective hospitalisations, and death during study period.

All data from summary cards and patient notes were entered by a pharmacist onto a Microsoft Access database held on a laptop computer, since some interpretation was occasionally required, and a knowledge of drugs was essential. For consistency the majority of data were entered by one research pharmacist.

Copies of all study prescription forms were obtained from the

Pharmacy Practice Division of the Common Services Agency (PPD). Drug acquisition costs excluding professional fees were calculated on the basis of figures in the Scottish Drug Tariff and the Chemist and Druggist.

Satisfaction measures The satisfaction of community pharmacists, general practitioners and patients with the new system was assessed by mailed questionnaires to each group. Questionnaire content was based on informed consensus from the project team, and interviews with selected study participants. Topics covered for community pharmacists and general practitioners included workload, satisfaction with the process, professional satisfaction, interprofessional communication, problems, remuneration and desirability of long-term implementation of the new system. Only general practitioners in the intervention group were surveyed.

Patients in both the control and intervention group were surveyed using a combination of factual questions and conjoint analysis. Information was obtained on direct and indirect costs associated with obtaining repeat prescriptions with factual questions. The technique of conjoint analysis was used to assess patient preference for the new system of obtaining their repeat prescriptions compared to traditional system. The technique is described in more detail in Chapter 4. Attributes identified from the interviews as important for the conjoint analysis were convenience, cost and clinical care.

Results

Demography

No statistical differences were identified in the proportion of fundholding, urban and rural practices, and number of general practitioner partners per practice in the control and intervention group practices. 1614 patients were recruited to the intervention group and 1460 patients were tagged in the control group of which 1405 patients were available for follow up; the remainder had died. Demography of the recruited patients is shown in Table 5.1.

Pharmacy collected patient care data

Compliance, adverse drug reactions/drug interactions, and other identified problems In total 153 compliance issues, 30 adverse drug reactions/drug interactions (mostly associated with NSAIDs or other

Table 5.1 Summary details of patients. (Modified with permission from Bond 1999.)

Summary details	Intervention	Control
Number of patients recruited	1614	1460
Male:female ratio	618:996	605:800
Male:female %	38%:62%	43%:57%
Number withdrawn	111	–
Mean number of items per patient	2.9	3.23

analgesiscs) and 68 other problems were identified by pharmacists (see Table 5.2).

There was great variation in the rate of detection of 'problems' by pharmacy. Table 5.3 shows the rate of pharmacy problem detection for the twenty pharmacies with more than 20 'registered' patients. The highest detection rate amongst the first 20 pharmacies was 50% indicating one 'problem' was detected for every two patients attending that pharmacy.

Table 5.2 Type and frequency of problems. (Modified with permission from Bond et al., 2000.)

Category of problem	Number of problems
Compliance problem	
Late to collect/ forgot/ not taking	47
Dose taken not the same as dose prescribed	34
Early to collect/taking too much	33
Items not required	24
Miscellaneous	10
Confused	5
Subtotal compliance	**153**
Adverse drug reactions	
Non steroidal anti-inflammatory drugs	8
Other analgesics	6
Miscellaneous	10
Drug interaction	
Prescription interaction	4
OTC interaction with prescribed drugs	2
Subtotal ADR/drug interaction	**30**
Other problems	
General symptoms	34
Drug related issues	15
Prescription problems	9
Miscellaneous	8
Problems related to study	2
Subtotal other problems	**68**

Table 5.3 Problems detected by pharmacy

Pharmacy	No. of patients	No. of compliance problems	(%)	No. of other problems	(%)	No. of ADR/DI	(%)	Total problems detected	Overall rate (%)
52	233	14	6.01	3	1.29	1	0.43	18	7.73
50	222	38	17.12	18	8.11	9	4.05	65	29.28
14	153	0	0.00	0	0.00	0	0.00	0	0.00
49	111	12	10.81	4	3.60	0	0.00	16	14.41
60	101	7	6.93	1	0.99	2	1.98	10	9.90
63	70	3	4.29	0	0.00	1	1.43	4	5.71
33	67	9	13.43	0	0.00	1	1.49	10	14.93
61	58	2	3.45	2	3.45	0	0.00	4	6.90
4	53	9	16.98	14	26.42	4	7.55	27	50.94
62	45	2	4.44	0	0.00	0	0.00	2	4.44
15	35	1	2.86	0	0.00	0	0.00	1	2.86
3	33	0	0.00	3	9.09	2	6.06	5	15.15
19	26	1	3.85	3	11.54	2	7.69	6	23.08
2	24	1	4.17	1	4.17	1	4.17	3	12.50
16	24	3	12.50	1	4.17	2	8.33	6	25.00
35	24	3	12.50	1	4.17	1	4.17	5	20.83
9	23	1	4.35	0	0.00	0	0.00	1	4.35
18	22	1	4.55	1	4.55	0	0.00	2	9.09
36	22	7	31.82	3	13.64	0	0.00	10	45.45

196 people had some sort of 'problem' identified, equivalent to 12% of the patients on the study. There was no correlation between the number or type of problem and the sex of the patient (see Table 5.4). Analysis of pharmacy detected problems according to general medical practice indicates there may be differences in the occurrence of such problems according to practices. However, an important confounding factor is the spread of patients across pharmacies. For example, one practice had a high occurrence of problems but the majority of these patients used one pharmacy which had a high problem-detection rate and may therefore have been more rigorous in following the protocol (see Table 5.5).

The mean number of items was calculated for each group subdivided according to the category of pharmacy detected problem. Those patients with a compliance problem or adverse drug reaction/interaction had a comparable number of prescribed items with the total intervention group. However, the mean number of items for those with other symptoms/problems was higher when compared to the intervention group as a whole (see Table 5.6).

Patient note search data

Data were collected on the number of drug compliance problems, adverse drug reactions and drug interactions detected by general practitioners in both the control and intervention groups through patient note searches. These are summarised in Table 5.5. Although the category 'other symptoms/problems' was collected this was not comparable to similar pharmacy data, due to the difficulties in defining 'other symptoms/problems'.

Overall, 2.5% of control group patients had a compliance problem and 6.7% had an ADR/DI detected by the general practitioner. In comparison, 1.4% of intervention patients had compliance problems and 6.7% had an ADR/DI detected by the general practitioner. Full details of the statistical comparison is published elsewhere (Bond *et al.*, 2000).

Examination of the data for patients with problems detected by the pharmacist compared to that for problems detected by the general practitioner indicated that only two patients with pharmacist-detected

Table 5.4 Pharmacy detected problems and patient sex

Sex	No of people	Compliance	DI/ADR	Other problem
f	996	81 (8.1%)	14 (1.4%)	44 (4.4%)
m	618	55 (8.9%)	8 (1.3%)	28 (4.5%)

Table 5.5 Numbers of problems detected by practice

Practice ID	Control or intervention	No. of notes searched	No. of compliance problems (C)	C %	No. of ADR/DI problems	ADR/DI %
10	Control	186	4	2.2	8	4.3
11	Control	116	3	2.6	16	13.8
22	Control	136	3	2.2	10	7.4
33	Control	172	3	1.7	9	5.2
44	Control	121	3	2.5	8	6.6
55	Control	135	1	0.7	5	3.7
66	Control	125	4	3.2	8	6.4
77	Control	114	4	3.5	4	3.5
88	Control	128	0	0	9	7.0
99	Control	172	10	5.8	17	9.9
Control total		1405	35	2.5	94	6.7
1	Intervention	99	2	2.0	11	11.1
2	Intervention	102	3	2.9	12	11.8
3	Intervention	108	0	0	1	0.9
4	Intervention	100	1	1.0	8	8.0
5	Intervention	100	3	3.0	10	10.0
6	Intervention	101	0	0	7	6.9
7	Intervention	104	1	1.0	5	4.8
8	Intervention	91	1	1.1	5	5.5
9	Intervention	100	2	2.0	2	2.0
Intervention total		905	13	1.4	61	6.7

Table 5.6 Mean number of items and number of patients with pharmacy detected problems

Category	No. of patients	Mean no. of items
Compliance	149	2.913
ADR/DI	30	3.033
Other problems	67	3.627
All intervention patients	1614	2.9

compliance problem were also noted by the general practitioner and only one patient with a pharmacist-detected ADR was also noted by the general practitioner. It was not clear from medical notes if a query from the pharmacist had brought these problems to the attention of the general practitioner. It can be concluded that the pharmacist is detecting different problems from the general practitioner.

The number of visits to the general practitioner was assessed. Although there appears to be a slightly higher number of total visits in the control group (average 6.722 per patient) compared to the intervention group (average 5.43 per patient), this was not statistically significant. Similarly, there was no difference in the death rate between control and intervention groups, which was 38 and 36 per 1000 patients respectively.

The number of non-elective hospital admissions was determined for each practice from patient medical notes. A slight difference is apparent between the control (57 per 1000 patients) and intervention groups (61 per 1000 patients) but this was not statistically significant.

Individual drug data

The total acquisition cost for all prescribed items is £369 020 (this represents 5374 items for 1555 patients).

The total acquisition cost for dispensed items is £302 034, and the total acquisition cost avoidance for non-dispensed items is £66 986, which represents 18.2% of all prescribed items. The number of patients who did not require their full prescribed quota of drugs was 1020 (i.e. 65.6% of the population analysed). Average 'savings' per patient not requiring their full prescribed quota of drugs therefore is £65.67 (and average annual 'saving' per patient overall would be £43).

The therapeutic group responsible for the largest proportion of prescribed and dispensed costs are the cardiovascular drugs. Drugs used to treat gastrointestinal problems represent the greatest area of 'savings', i.e. largest proportion of non-dispensed costs.

Satisfaction

Pharmacists   A response was received from 36 pharmacies. These respondents had 1226 patients between them representing 75% of the total number of intervention patients.

28.6% of respondents were male and 61.2% female. The majority of respondents (46.9%) were from small multiples with 28.6% single pharmacy outlets and 14.3% large multiples.

36.7% of respondents felt the study had improved their relationship with study patients and only 8.2% felt their relationship had worsened. It was suggested that the study gave pharmacists an 'excuse' to speak to patients and ask about medication without appearing 'nosy'.

The professional relationship with general practitioners, practice managers and receptionists appeared largely unaffected by the study.

Interview and discussion group data indicated that there was a split in pharmacists' opinion of which type of patient benefited most from the study system. Patients on simple medication regimens were cited as being most suitable because there was less likelihood of medication being changed which could cause confusion. However, this group of patients was less likely to require pharmacist input. Correspondingly, patients on more complex medication regimens may benefit more in terms of quality of care but these patients are more prone to confusion and more time-consuming to manage.

Feedback from interviews/discussions indicated that there may have been a change in the distribution of repeat prescription requests with the dispensing workload being spread more evenly throughout the day and week (more on Saturdays). Questionnaire results indicated that 63.3% of respondents did not believe there was such a change, with 26.5% believing there was. This illustrates the complementary relationship between quantitative and qualitative data.

General practices   Of the 35 questionnaires distributed to the intervention general practitioners, 33 were returned (94%) (see Table 5.7).

Significantly more general practitioners stated that they would prefer to provide a new type of repeat prescribing system for their patients (χ^2 p = <0.001), of these significantly more chose to modify the system rather than to continue with the study system per se (χ^2 p = <0.01).

Statistical association between questions could not be demonstrated due to the small sample size. Likewise, differences between surgeries, and city versus non-city locations could not be shown.

Of the 20 questionnaires distributed to practice managers, 100% were returned, including a reply from a practice that had split from an intervention practice during the study. More than half of the practice managers stated that they would prefer to provide a new type of repeat prescribing system for their patients, and of these most would choose a modification of the study system.

Patients   High patient satisfaction with the new system was shown by 81% of patients in the intervention group who stated a preference for the new method of obtaining repeat medicines compared to their previous traditional system. If non-returned questionnaires indicated dissatisfaction (the worst case scenario), preference for the new repeat system would drop to 58%.

Table 5.7 General practitioner replies to satisfaction questionnaire

Question		%	(n)
Compared to your traditional repeat system, do you think that you review your study patients' medication more or less often?	More often	42	(33)
	The same	42	
	Less often	15	
Have you found the designated patient repeat medicine review appointments useful?	Yes	63	(32)
	No	38	
Do you think that the pharmacist's input during the study has improved the quality of medication control provided for any of your patients?	Yes	30	(33)
	Unsure	52	
	No	18	
Do you think that the pharmacist's input during the study has worsened the quality of medication control provided for any of your patients?	Yes	–	(33)
	Unsure	24	
	No	76	
Overall, do you think that the study has altered your professional relationship with the pharmacist?	Yes, improved	21	(33)
	Yes, worsened	3	
	No	76	
Would you like any study patients to continue with the repeat prescribing system in your practice?	Yes	75	(32)
	No	25	
Would you like to extend this repeat prescribing system to additional patients in your practice, not currently in the study?	Yes	59	(32)
	No	41	
Which system of repeat prescribing would you prefer to provide for your patients?	Study system	19	(32)
	Traditional system	19	
	Modified version of the study system	63[a]	
	Don't mind	–	

[a] χ^2 p < 0.01

Increased preference for the new repeat system was apparent if patients realised a time or cost saving. Preference for the new system was also greater when advice had been offered by the community pharmacist, with virtually all patients finding the advice helpful. However, patients did not indicate that the advice given on the new system was any greater than that they had received whilst using the traditional repeat method. The level of pharmaceutical advice and counselling may have already been high or, alternatively, it may not have been appropriate to offer advice or counselling.

The majority of patients commented on the favourable convenience and financial aspects of the system, a large number also felt reassured that the pharmacist was taking an interest in their medication and felt that he/she was a 'safety net' for the general practitioner. An increase in reassurance can be considered as an increase in quality of healthcare. The concept of increased quality of healthcare was asked in the pilot and appeared to be misunderstood by many respondents and for this reason was omitted from the final questionnaire.

Patients showed greater satisfaction on visiting their general practitioner less often regarding repeat prescriptions. Comments indicated that this was due to increased convenience, particularly by those in full-time employment. It had been thought that some patients may value visiting their general practitioner for health reassurance, a role which may have been taken over by the pharmacist in the study.

Details of the traditional repeat method which intervention patients had used prior to the study did not appear to influence patient preference for the new system. Journey time, bus fare and car mileage were not associated with satisfaction, which suggests that time and cost savings influenced satisfaction, through decreased visits to the surgery irrespective of journey length or cost.

Lower preference for the new system was shown if the patient had not always obtained their medicines from the same pharmacy, if they previously received more than one month's medication on prescription, or if they had run out previously. The group who had run out of medicines on the traditional system may have done so because of confusion or disorganisation, in which case the new method would not have been an advantage to them.

The conjoint analysis identified that convenience was particularly important to the intervention group whilst cost was important to both control and intervention groups.

Implications for practice

Evidence of study

The limitations of the study should first be acknowledged. Practices were asked to recruit 250 patients at a rate of 25 patients per week over a ten-week period and a protocol for patient recruitment was provided. The recruitment population was all patients who currently receive medication on repeat prescription and did not come under the exclusion criteria. The intention was to cover all ages and disease states so there should not have been any selection of patients by general practitioners. However, selection may have taken place in two ways: first the receptionist may not have noted patients' names down on the recruitment list if they knew they came under the exclusion criteria; secondly, the general practitioner may have decided for reasons outwith the protocol that a patient was not suitable.

In theory, such patient selection may have affected the study patient sample and subsequently the results. A tendency to select patients on a straightforward medication regimen would reduce the likelihood of pharmacy intervention, affect the patient care outcome measures and minimise the apparent 'value added' impact of the system.

The study clearly demonstrated that the more formal involvement of community pharmacists in the repeat prescribing/dispensing process allowed identification of compliance problems, adverse drug reactions, drug interactions and other drug-related problems.

The health economic implications of these observations were not formally explored but the possible cost avoidance of hospital admission, for example due to a gastrointestinal bleed associated with NSAID use, qualitatively supports potential health economic benefits.

Data were collected from patient notes on the number of medication review visits, but this proved extremely difficult due to the subjective nature of determining what actually was a review visit. For this reason we have considered only the total number of visits, assuming that visits for other reasons, e.g. acute problems, should be comparable in the control and intervention group. There was no difference in the total number of visits to the general practitioner between the groups. It was anticipated that intervention group patients might go to their general practitioner slightly more often than the control group because of the enforced medical review (assuming that control group patients are reviewed less frequently).

There are indications from the study results that there could be significant cost avoidance associated with the new system, mostly due to non-dispensed prescribed medication, but also due to early additional identification of drug-related problems. The full significance of these aspects was beyond the scope of this current study. A detailed study would need to consider the nature of drugs not dispensed and the possible resultant clinical implications of these drugs not being taken as intended. This would have to be balanced against the 'saving' attributable to the non-dispensing.

We can speculate on how this system could be incorporated into normal practice. Pharmacists could be contracted locally to provide a repeat prescription monitoring service by health boards or fundholding practices, or such a system could be negotiated centrally as part of the pharmacist's remuneration package.

The type of patient suitable for such a repeat system requires consideration. Patients on stable, straightforward medication regimens are the easiest to administer at a practice and pharmacy level and feedback from both practice and pharmacy (as reported elsewhere) indicated that these patients are preferred. Patients who are not stable and require changes to medication take up more time for both the pharmacy and practice. However, such patients may experience more benefit from the system. The repeat prescribing study requires the pharmacist to take on board increased responsibility for repeat prescriptions. Although general practitioners may be in agreement for patients on regular therapy to be managed in this way they may not be so keen to relinquish responsibility for patients taking less straightforward medication.

The study system evolved as a way of allowing community pharmacists to monitor and authorise repeat prescriptions under the current system. The study demonstrated the feasibility of the principle and did not recommend that the mechanism per se be continued due to resultant reimbursement and remuneration issues for community pharmacists. A robust system for delivery of the services now needs to be developed which will allow prompt payment to the community pharmacist at each dispensing. Recent White Papers (Scottish Health Service Management Executive, 1997; Secretary of State for Scotland, 1997) explicitly highlight the potential for pharmacy to become increasingly involved and integrated within the primary healthcare team, and mechanisms for remunerating such new roles are currently being developed.

The future

Studies elsewhere, particularly in Tayside and Dorset, have similarly demonstrated the feasibility and benefit of involving pharmacists in managing repeat prescribing. On the basis of these studies, the study described in this chapter and Chapter 6, and those mentioned in Chapter 10, there are a range of models of pharmacy input to general practice prescribing. The most basic of these, which could be implemented immediately by all pharmacists, based on the system described in this chapter. The most proactive model would be one in which the pharmacist could operate within the general practice setting, reviewing patient notes and making clinical recommendations to general practitioners to improve the care of their patients. This would be similar to the pharmacy input described in Chapter 6.

In order further to quantify the benefits of involving pharmacists, the Department of Health awarded funding to a range of pilot repeat prescribing projects in 1997. The biggest of these was delivered by a consortium led by the National Pharmaceutical Association, including the Pharmaceutical Services Negotiating Committee, the University of York, and ourselves at the University of Aberdeen. The outcome of these projects is keenly awaited, and it is hoped it will be instrumental in supporting a change of regulation that would formally allow pharmacy a greater role in this regard.

Similarly, the Crown review of Supply, Distribution and Administration of Medicines has recommended a limited deregulation of NHS prescribing, extending prescribing rights to a range of professionals under specific circumstances (Crown, 1999). It may be that the recommendations of this committee could also facilitate a formal role for community pharmacy endorsed by statute.

Finally, the electronic age is with us! Information technology (IT) has revolutionised many aspects of life in the developed world and tasks as varied as booking a holiday or managing finances are all managed via computer networks that link involved stakeholders. In addition, many individuals worldwide communicate via the internet and email, which links a diversity of hardware and software systems. To date the NHS has failed to optimise the potential of IT fully, although individual service providers, or professional groupings, have increasingly developed their own specialised systems. The need for these systems to be compatible and allow data interchange has been officially recognised in the recent White Paper 'Designed to Care', which highlights the objective of linking general practice surgeries and secondary care through the NHS net. This should allow speedy patient data transfer to improve the service currently offered across the primary-secondary care interface. However, no official mention is made of extending the net to include either community pharmacy or the Pharmacy Practice Division, which has responsibility for prescription pricing, providing information to inform the reimbursement of community pharmacists for drugs which they have dispensed against NHS prescriptions, and providing feedback to general practitioners, dentists and nurse prescribers on the drugs which they have prescribed as indicated by the prescriptions which have been dispensed.

There currently appears to be an unwritten policy which indicates a will to involve community pharmacy in the second wave of the NHS net. In anticipation of this, the Royal Pharmaceutical Society of Great Britain produced an information strategy for pharmacy as part of its Pharmacy in a New Age initiative. The strategy focused on ways in which IT could be used to enhance the availability of information to pharmacists, patients and the public, and recognised the requirement for pharmacists to have access to electronically held patient information owned by other professionals.

If electronic links were developed which allowed community pharmacy and general practice to talk to each other, the potential for community pharmacists' clinical input into a wide range of prescribing services would be greatly enhanced. Access to patient records from the 'high street', at levels of access agreed with both general practitioners and patients, would allow pharmacists to make informed decisions about therapy, without leaving their premises, thus overcoming some of the barriers to greater primary healthcare team involvement experienced at the moment, and maintaining pharmacists' much highlighted accessibility to the public.

Acknowledgements

We gratefully acknowledge the participation of all professionals (community pharmacists, general practitioners and general practice staff) and patients. Without them this study would not have been possible. Further details of the study can be found in Bond *et al.* (2000) and Jones *et al.* (2000). We also acknowledge the support of Grampian Health Board in funding this study under the Primary Care Development Fund.

Notes

1. Whilst the NHS sum for the payment of pharmaceutical services 'the Global sum' is fixed, and increases are negotiated annually, the mechanism for distributing the sum uses the prescription volume of individual contractors. This is not to say that pharmacists are only required to dispense prescriptions, as their wider role is acknowledged and specified in the Code of Ethics, but this mechanism for remuneration sometimes results in a perception that payment is based on an item of service, namely the dispensed prescription.

2. Whilst the Medicines Act allows repeat dispensing this is not generally reflected in the NHS regulations A variation primarily to allow drugs of misuse to be dispensed in instalments within a total period of 14 days has been introduced in Scotland and is described in the Scottish Drug Tarriff 1996. It has become accepted practice to allow prescriptions in excess of the 14 days stipulated to be dispensed, mainly as weekly instalments in monitored dosage systems for nursing homes. Lack of clarity in the regulations has restricted the widespread use of the regulation in other circumstances.

References

Anonymous (1992a). Puzzling prescription. *Pharm J* 248: 224.
Anonymous (1992b). Mystical prescription. *Pharm J* 249: 593.
Anonymous (1992c). Physical prescription. *Pharm J* 249: 258.
Bond C M (1999). Pharamcy and primary health care. In: Sims J, ed. *Primary Health Care Sciences*. London: Whurr.
Bond C M, Hickey F, Matheson C (1997). Problems and pitfalls in practice research. *Pharm J* 258: 12–13.
Bond C M, Matheson C I, Williams S, *et al.* (2000). Repeat Prescribing: a role for community pharmacists in monitoring and controlling repeat prescriptions. *Br J Gen Pract* 50: 271–5.
Bond C M, Sinclair H K, Taylor R J, *et al.* (1995). Pharmacists: a resource for general practice? *Int J Pharm Pract* 3: 85–90.
Bond C M, Taylor R J, Williams A, *et al.* (1993). *The role of the pharmacist in encouraging high quality prescribing.* Report to Grampian Health Board on research project grant.
Crown J (1999). *Review of the prescribing, supply and administration of medicines.* London: Department of Health.
Department of Health (1987). Promoting better health *Government White Paper* CM 249. London: HMSO.
Department of Health (1999). *Protecting and using patient information.* A manual for Caldicott guardians. Edinburgh: The Scottish Office.
Department of Health and Royal Pharmaceutical Society of Great Britain (1992). *Pharmaceutical Care: The future for community pharmacy.* Joint Working Party on the future role of the community pharmaceutical services.
Government White Paper (1996). *Primary care: choice and opportunity.* London: HMSO.
Harris C M, Dajda R (1996). The scale of repeat prescribing. *Br J Gen Pract*: 46: 649–53.
Irish Pharmaceutical Contractors Committee (1996). Clause 9 of agreement on the future provision and improvement of community pharmacy services under the Health Act 1970. Irish Pharmaceutical Union.
Jones J, Matheson C I, Bond C M (2000). Patients' satisfaction with a novel system of repeat prescribing. Submitted to *Int J Pharm Pract.*
National Audit Office (1993). *Repeat prescribing by general medical practitioners in England.* Report by the Comptroller and Auditor General. London: HMSO 897.
National Audit Office (1994). *A prescription for improvement.* Report by the Comptroller and Auditor General. London: HMSO.

Scottish Health Service Management Executive (1997). *Primary Care: agenda for action*. Edinburgh: Scottish Office Department of Health.

Scottish Office (1993). *Accountability reviews: priorities and planning guidance*. The Scottish Office NHS MEL 155.

Secretary of State for Scotland (1997). *Designed to care: reviewing the National Health Service in Scotland* Cm 3811. Edinburgh: Scottish Office Department of Health.

Spencer J A, Edwards C (1992). Pharmacy beyond the dispensary: general practitioners' views. *BMJ* 304: 1670–72.

Zermansky A G (1996). Who controls repeats? *Br J Gen Pract* 46: 643–47.

6

Disease management

Sheena Macgregor

Introduction

Disease management systems have the potential to benefit patients, provided they can deliver improved continuity of care, decrease inappropriate treatment and encourage more effective interventions. The concept appeals to policy makers because it attempts to maximise cost effectiveness while improving quality of care and patient satisfaction. However, if a disease management approach is to be successful it needs to be patient-centred, outcome focused, evidence-based, credible, and sufficiently flexible to account for patient individuality. It also needs to take into consideration cost, professional consensus on clinical practice, availability of local facilities and acceptability to patients if implementation in the 'real world' is to be achievable.

Successful implementation of a disease management approach to patient care would be incompatible with traditional doctor-centred practice. However, developments in the structure, function and funding of primary care services in recent years have contributed to organisational changes in general practice. There is greater emphasis on teamwork and appropriate skill mix, which has resulted in expansion of primary care multidisciplinary teams, with the aim of achieving a more cost-effective and patient-centred service. The result is increased community-based care for chronic disease management. Implementation of a quality system of patient care requires all of the multidisciplinary team members who contribute to that care sharing information on desired outcomes and on the consequences of treatment. They need to work together in an organised system to deliver defined patient outcomes. Multidisciplinary care pathways of this kind rarely feature in the primary care setting and where GPs, nurses and professions allied to medicine (PAMs) provide care packages without pharmacist input, medication-related issues are often unidentified and their importance overlooked. Care pathways promote collaboration and communication among members of the healthcare team and reduce unnecessary variation in the management of patients. They also ensure that all patients receive consistent high quality care by the most appropriate team member, with each member having a clearly defined role and understanding the contribution of the other members in the overall plan. They focus on the needs of the patient, minimising territorial issues between team members and allowing them to concentrate on improving quality of care. Within such a team the pharmacist would be expected to have a responsibility to ensure that drug treatment and related care issues are identified and addressed.

The move to a more patient-centred approach to disease management also requires an understanding of how the patient perceives his illness and its treatment. Patients obtain information about their medicines from a wide range of sources, including family and friends, the media and, increasingly, the internet, in addition to healthcare professionals. Pharmacists can facilitate patient compliance with medication, provide support to patients and their carers and promote evidence-based prescribing to ensure appropriate utilisation of medicines by the healthcare team. Importantly, they can also ensure that information provided by the healthcare team is consistent and accurate. It must be remembered that evidence-based medicine is generated from carefully defined populations, while daily practice involves dealing with individual patients. There is no value in offering evidence-based treatment unless the patient is willing to accept it and without their co-operation we cannot achieve a successful outcome. Patients need to be involved in deciding on the most suitable treatment options so that a concordant decision is achieved.

Disease management systems aim to achieve the best outcomes for disease using a combination of clinical evidence, patient education, appropriate consultations and appropriate use of medicines, all co-ordinated by a case manager. Development of locally agreed protocols based on evidence-based guidelines is fundamental to achieving this. However, provision of information alone is rarely sufficient to stimulate corresponding changes in practice (Grol, 1992; Wensing *et al.*, 1998). Considerable effort is directed towards developing guidelines based on good research and clinical experience. This is increasingly seen as an essential tool for achieving high quality care. However, little attention has been given as to how implementation can be achieved at patient level. A local protocol may ensure that new disease presentations are treated appropriately but full guideline implementation requires a systematic review of patients already receiving treatment. This can be a time consuming process involving identification of patients, review of medical case notes, discussion with the individual patients to explain why changes are recommended and to agree treatment plans, follow up and monitoring. The pharmacist not only has the necessary skills to facilitate implementation of disease management guidelines at practice level, to audit clinical practice and to educate patients on medicine compliance and lifestyle, but to identify pharmaceutical care issues which may be unrelated to the current medical problem. Since patients rarely fit into single disease categories, the importance of this unique skill cannot be over emphasised. Furthermore the pharmacist's potential ability to select medicines and dosage for individual patients from agreed protocols following medical diagnosis or assessment has been identified, and consensus is that it should be promoted.

In the US, pharmacists have been moving towards integration into family practitioner teams since the mid-1970s (Perry and Hurley, 1975; Brown *et al.*, 1979; Hart *et al.*, 1979; Haxby, *et al.* 1988). Since then pharmacist-led clinics based in primary care have been established (Furmega, 1993; Coast-Senior *et al.*, 1998). More recently, disease management has reached the community pharmacy setting (Lima, 1998). However, little has been documented in the UK prior to 1990. Since then pharmacy practice development has been largely influenced by the application of the concept of 'pharmaceutical care' (Hepler and Strand, 1990). Pharmaceutical care is a systematic, rational and comprehensive approach to drug therapy decisions. It offers the pharmacist a patient-centred philosophy of practice that makes the identification, resolution and prevention of drug therapy problems the responsibility of the practitioner. The practice of pharmaceutical care is focused on ensuring that all drug therapy is appropriate, effective, safe and convenient. It must therefore be comprehensive and cannot focus entirely on one disease at a time if a reduction in drug-related morbidity and mortality is to be achieved (Cipolle *et al.*, 1998).

Using the example of peptic ulcer disease, this chapter aims to illustrate the features of a systematic approach to care, with a pharmacist co-ordinating disease management. The intention of this study was to introduce a system that would allow a multidisciplinary team approach to contribute to the evidence-based, patient focused, economically rational management of dyspepsia that makes best use of public funds and enhances the quality of life for the patient. Secondly, the study assessed whether such a model could provide a framework for pharmacist management of other chronic disease states.

Research questions

In 1994/95, the cost to the National Health Service in Scotland of medicines used to treat upper gastrointestinal disorders, including gastric and
duodenal ulcer, reflux oesophagitis and non-ulcer dyspepsia, was £61
million. This represents 14.7% of the cost of all medicines prescribed in
general practice (Pharmacy Practice Division, Edinburgh, personal communication). Additionally, 30–40% of patients receive these medicines
on repeat prescription without having a firm diagnosis. Apart from
reduction in quality of life for these patients, there are considerable
financial implications for their management. Costs are rising since the
introduction of the proton-pump inhibitors (PPIs) and it is doubtful
whether continuing this scale of drug expenditure for patients without
a confirmed diagnosis, often to compensate for poor lifestyle, can be
justified.

Evidence-based recommendations for the management of dyspepsia have changed in recent years. *Helicobacter pylori* (*H. pylori*) infection occurs in over 70% of patients with gastric ulcer (Barnes, 1995) and
in over 90% of patients with duodenal ulcer (Axon, 1993). Evidence is
also accumulating which indicates that early *Helicobacter* eradication
may be beneficial. *H. pylori* has been established as the causative organ-
ism in duodenal ulcer and eradication of the bacteria reduces the annual
relapse rate to 0–3%, compared to 60–90% for untreated patients, and
10–30% for patients maintained on histamine H_2-receptor antagonists
(H_2RAs) (Hawkey, 1994). This new approach offers two potential
advantages over long-term maintenance therapy. First, the quality of life
for patients can be improved and, secondly, the cost of management
should be reduced as low re-infection and relapse rates reduce the need
for ulcer healing drugs. A Scottish Home and Health Department
Accountability Review (1993) targeted treatment of upper gastrointestinal disorders as a priority area for prescribing review. The
National Institute of Health (NIH) Consensus Panel (1994) also recommended that patients with gastric or duodenal ulcers who were infected
with *H. pylori* should be treated with antimicrobial agents.

An audit of the patients in Downfield Surgery in Dundee, where
the author was a Clinical Pharmacist, revealed that 7% of the total practice population (456 patients) were prescribed repeat H_2RAs or PPIs at
a cost of £68 000 (12% of the medicines budget). Of these patients, 37%
(173 patients) had no endoscopically or radiologically proven diagnosis
but the drugs which they received were costing the practice £25 000 per
annum; 6% had proven history of gastric ulcer, 27% of duodenal ulcer

and 29% of gastro-oesophageal reflux disease. These findings are in line with other practices in Tayside (Goudie *et al.*, 1996).

Partners at Downfield Surgery were in agreement that treatment of upper gastrointestinal disease should be diagnosis-based. However, detailed review of patients on long-term medication is time consuming. Where *H. pylori* eradication is undertaken, patient compliance is essential for a successful outcome. Unpleasant side effects are likely to result in patients failing to complete the course unless time is taken to explain to patients what they can expect and the importance of strict compliance. Again, this has time implications. Most general practitioners are already over-stretched, but the input of pharmacists to rational and cost-effective prescribing, coupled with their ability to educate patients on medicines compliance and lifestyle, makes them ideally placed to manage review of these patients within previously agreed guidelines. Our approach was therefore to build on the experience gained from pharmacist-led anticoagulant clinics (Macgregor *et al.*, 1996) and neurogenic pain management and to evaluate the benefits and costs of running a pharmacist-managed clinic to review patients prescribed repeat ulcer-healing agents.

The research question addressed by this study can therefore be expressed as follows: 'Does a diagnosis-based, treatment protocol approach to the eradication of *Helicobacter pylori* utilising a pharmacist-managed clinic, provide a beneficial approach to the management of upper gastrointestinal disease in general practice?'

This translates into the aim of the study, which was to develop, implement and assess the costs and benefits of a pharmacist-led clinic to manage the care of patients with upper gastrointestinal disease.

Method

Patient selection

Patients prescribed ulcer-healing medicines on repeat prescription were identified using computerised practice records. Their medical case notes were then reviewed jointly by the pharmacist and a GP. Patients who had no recorded diagnosis and had not requested a prescription in the last six months had the H_2RA or PPI discontinued to ensure that any future requirement for ulcer healing medication would necessitate a general practitioner consultation. Elderly patients receiving non-steroidal anti-inflammatory drugs (NSAIDs) and other patients, who in the clinical judgement of the general practitioner should continue therapy, were also excluded. The remaining patients were invited to attend a pharmacist-managed clinic for review in accordance with a protocol previously agreed with the general practitioners. In the absence of published research in primary care, the protocol devised was based on the available literature, and in consultation with general practitioners in the practice and local gastroenterologists. It has since been modified on a number of occasions in line with the continually changing evidence base.

The practice aim is for all future patients with upper gastrointestinal disorders to be treated according to diagnosis. Patients who attended a general practitioner with symptoms of dyspepsia for the first time were therefore prescribed four weeks of simple antacid therapy and given lifestyle advice, unless symptoms indicating urgent management necessitated early endoscopy. Patients who remained symptomatic on antacids were referred to the pharmacist clinic for further management.

Patient screening

Documentation for use in the clinic was developed. This was designed to record current symptoms, relevant past medical history, current prescribed and over-the-counter (OTC) medication and drug allergies. It was then used to identify unrelated pharmaceutical care issues, and to record outcomes and the management care plan agreed with the patient. This was inserted into patients' case notes following attendance at the clinic.

Helicobacter pylori status

Helicobacter pylori status was determined initially using a commercially available serological testing kit (Helisal). Unless a diagnosis was recorded in the notes, patients with a negative result were referred for endoscopy and testing for *campylobacter*-like organisms (CLO). This standard procedure, known as 'biopsy urease', is based on urease activity of the *Helicobacter pylori* bacteria releasing ammonia measured by an observed colour change in the reagent from yellow to pink. This ensured that future drug treatment was diagnosis based. Four weeks after treatment [13]carbon urea breath testing (UBT) was carried out by practice nurses to determine eradication success or failure.

Controversy surrounds the accuracy of near patient serological test kits (Anonymous, 1997). They are neither 100% specific or sensitive for *H. pylori*. [13]Carbon urea breath tests, although simple to perform in the general practitioner surgery, have to be sent for external analysis and do not allow an instantaneous decision to be made in the clinic setting. At the time of the study these tests were available only on a named patient basis. CLO tests involve a surgical procedure and are inappropriate for primary care use. Breath tests and CLO biopsies were therefore reserved for patients with alarm symptoms and for patient follow-up, where serological testing is inappropriate due to continued circulation of autoantibodies in blood for up to a year (Kosunen *et al.*, 1992)

Endoscopy referral

Evidence in secondary care indicates that all patients over 45 years presenting with dyspepsia for the first time should have gastroscopy, because of the need to exclude significant disease such as gastric carcinoma. However, the general practitioners in the practice argued convincingly that age was only one of a number of factors to be considered when assessing a patient, and that it was inappropriate to routinely investigate all patients on the basis of age alone. Referral was therefore confined to new patients with symptoms of concern, and patients who remained symptomatic following successful eradication of *H. pylori*.

Eradication therapy

Patients with a positive *H. pylori* result were prescribed appropriate eradication therapy, depending on co-existing diseases and interacting medicines. Triple therapy (omeprazole 40 mg daily, amoxicillin 1 g twice daily and metronidazole 400 mg three times daily) for seven days was prescribed first line with dual therapy (omeprazole 40 mg daily and clarithromycin 500 mg three times daily) for 14 days as second line. In patients with active duodenal ulcers, omeprazole was continued for a further seven days. Patients with a history of bleeding ulcers were maintained on an H_2RA until eradication was confirmed. Patients remaining positive for *H. pylori* were prescribed a further, different, course of eradication therapy.

A variety of triple therapy regimens for seven days form the basis of current recommended options. Dual therapy requiring 14 days' treatment was the alternative second line therapy adopted in this study. The extended duration, reduced efficacy and increased potential for non-compliance by the patient has resulted in this treatment being superseded by alternative triple therapy regimens (Tytgat, 1994). Quadruple therapies, which may allow shorter courses and increased patient acceptability, are being developed (De Boer *et al.*, 1997; Kung *et al.*, 1997) and it is likely that therapy recommendations will continue to change over the next few years.

Patient counselling

Patients were counselled by the pharmacist, with regard to potential side effects of the eradication medicines, and the need to complete the course. They were also advised that symptom relief may not be instantaneous following treatment, but may take several weeks for maximum improvement to be realised. All patients were given lifestyle advice. Warning regarding the alcohol-metronidazole interaction was given where appropriate, and women prescribed the combined oral contraceptive pill were advised to use alternative contraception. Patient information leaflets were distributed to back up oral information and patients were encouraged to telephone for advice rather than to stop treatment if they were experiencing problems.

Economic analysis

Case notes were reviewed after six months to identify patients who continued to require management of upper gastrointestinal disease. The Pharmacoeconomic Research Centre at St Andrews University carried out economic analysis for the undiagnosed patients and for new patients. The data collected were used to structure a series of decision trees on which the cost minimisation analysis was based, for each of the patient groups. The analysis was performed using Decision Program Language (DPL) software from Applied Decision Analysis Inc., Memlo, California, USA.

Results

Patients without an endoscopically or radiologically confirmed diagnosis

Of the 173 patients without a diagnosis, repeat medication was discontinued in 67 patients (39%) who requested repeat prescriptions intermittently and had not done so for at least six months. Forty-four patients (25%) were continued on their ulcer-healing medicines, 29 due to disabling concurrent medical problems, six in view of advancing age and a further nine on NSAIDs for whom cover with an H_2RA was considered to be necessary.

The remaining 62 patients (36%) were invited to attend the clinic. One patient refused to attend and had his medication discontinued.

Maintenance therapy costs for the remaining 61 patients was £14 061 per annum. Of these patients, 52 (85%) were positive for H. *pylori*. Two patients refused to take eradication therapy, one because of prescription charges, the second because he could not afford to risk symptoms which might result in having to be absent from work and which he had experienced on a previous occasion. Of the 50 patients who accepted eradication therapy, 44 (88%) achieved successful eradication with the first regimen. The remaining six patients (12%) were successful after a second-line regimen. Following eradication of H. *pylori*, eight patients continued to have symptoms of dyspepsia and were referred for endoscopy. Of these, two were recommenced on the same medication as prior to eradication therapy, three were maintained on less expensive regimens. Three patients were diagnosed as having Barrett's oesophagitis and were commenced on proton pump inhibitors.

Of the nine patients who tested negative for H. *pylori*, four were referred for endoscopy, one was delayed pending unrelated surgery and four refused this procedure. Of those scoped, three were diagnosed as having gastro-oesophageal reflux disease and one gastritis/duodenitis. Seven of the nine patients who tested negative were continued on maintenance therapy in accordance with the local protocol.

Within the practice the overall cost of post-H. *pylori* eradication maintenance therapy was reduced from £14 061 to £2851 per annum. The total cost of the eradication process amounted to £4400 for these patients.

Patients with no previous diagnosis presenting with dyspepsia for the first time

Fifty-eight patients with no previous history of upper gastrointestinal disease attended the clinic and were tested for H. *pylori*. Thirty-seven (64%) tested positive. One refused therapy due to prescription costs but did not continue to take antacid therapy either.

Of the patients who tested H. *pylori* positive, 34 did not require long-term medication. Thirty patients had the infection eradicated successfully after the first attempt and a further six at the second-line regimen. The two patients who remained symptomatic despite successful eradication of the bacteria agreed to be referred for endoscopy, which showed gastro-oesophageal reflux disease requiring maintenance with Gaviscon. The total cost of the eradication procedure for this group of patients amounted to £3298.

Of the 21 H. *pylori*-negative patients, five were referred for endoscopy (at a total cost of £685) which revealed diagnoses of gastritis (one), Barrett's oesophagitis (two) and no abnormality in three. Five further patients refused this procedure. The remaining eleven did not feel it necessary at this stage, symptoms having resolved with antacid, and a decision was made to carry out endoscopy should there be a recurrence (McIntyre *et al.*, 1997).

Patients with a history of duodenal or gastric ulcer

A total of 94 patients with an endoscopically or radiologically confirmed diagnosis of duodenal ulcer (85) or gastric ulcer (nine) were identified. Cost of existing maintenance therapy was £19 322 per annum for patients with duodenal ulceration and £1720 for patients with gastric ulceration. Seventy of the duodenal ulcer patients and all nine of the gastric ulcer patients were positive for *H. pylori*.

Of the nine gastric ulcer patients, seven had the infection eradicated successfully with the first regimen, the remaining two with the second-line regimen. None of these patients required post-eradication maintenance therapy.

Sixty *H. pylori*-positive patients with a history of duodenal ulcer were successfully eradicated following the first drug regimen, a further eight patients following a second regimen. Two patients refused eradication therapy. Four of these patients who were successfully eradicated (two with co-existing gastro-oesophageal reflux disease) have required maintenance therapy.

Only 70 out of the 85 duodenal ulcer patients (82%) were identified as being *H. pylori*-positive by serological testing. Since studies have shown 95% of duodenal ulcer patients to be *H. pylori*-positive, it is likely that serological testing has been insufficiently sensitive to detect all the infected duodenal ulcer patients. For these patients the opportunity to reduce doses of medication to maintenance levels was taken meantime, although UBT may be undertaken to confirm *H. pylori* status in the future.

The cost of maintenance therapy post-*H. pylori* eradication reduced to £3980 for patients with a history of duodenal ulcer and £312 for gastric ulcer, representing a total cost reduction of £16 750 per annum, assuming these patients would have continued to take maintenance therapy. The total cost of the eradication process amounted to £6534 for these patients.

Cost benefit analysis

Pharmacoeconomists evaluated costs and outcomes for new patients and patients without a confirmed diagnosis. The aim of decision analysis is to arrive at the expected total cost per patient. The expected cost of an option is calculated by summing the products of the probability of occurrence and the cost of each of its sub-branches (Craig *et al.*, 1996). Depending on the objective of the decision-maker, the option with the highest expected value would then be selected as the most likely method of achieving the most desirable outcome, or in this case the lowest expected cost. The majority of patients tested were found to be *H. pylori*-positive and responded successfully to eradication therapy with no further symptoms and no recurrence of problems, and therefore with no further associated costs.

The decision tree for new patients was based on a comparison of our strategy versus conventional empirical treatment, using published treatment algorithms (McIntyre *et al.*, 1997). In patients aged less than 45, the algorithm of treatment was based on the study by Briggs *et al.* (1996) whereby a course of cimetidine 800 mg per day for four weeks was given, achieving healing rates of 80%. If, at the end of the course, symptoms recurred, a second course was prescribed and, for those patients whose symptoms persisted beyond eight weeks after the first course of cimetidine, it was assumed that long-term maintenance treatment would be required. For patients aged 45 or over, the algorithm of Hallissey *et al.* (1990) whereby all patients presenting for the first time were referred for endoscopy, was used. Seventy-five percent of all these patients required maintenance therapy following endoscopic diagnosis. Decision analysis for new patients determined the expected total cost per patient with and without *H. pylori* eradication treatment. To continue therapy over a new patient's expected life span was calculated at £384 but the cost if tested and treated accordingly was calculated at £200, a saving of £184.

The decision tree analysis for patients already prescribed repeat ulcer healing medicines but without a confirmed diagnosis, also indicated that it would probably be financially beneficial to test for *H. pylori* and to treat accordingly, with a saving of £2191 for each undiagnosed patient.

Discussion

The treatment of upper gastrointestinal disorders represents a significant workload and has major financial implications in primary care. Control of the problem can be achieved through structured review of patients with chronic complaints and adherence to systems to manage those presenting with symptoms for the first time. As a result expenditure on ulcer-healing medicines for the study practice is reducing at a time when it is increasing throughout Scotland as a whole.

Patients without an endoscopically or radiologically confirmed diagnosis

This group of patients has not been addressed by any of the recently published guidelines, yet they present a problem of considerable clinical and economical importance.

Simple decision analysis, as discussed in this chapter, suggests that when a general practitioner is faced with a number of patients with no diagnosis but receiving maintenance therapy, it would probably be financially beneficial if these patients were tested for *H. pylori* and treated accordingly. The data from this study suggest that the number of patients who are infected with *H. pylori* bacteria, and who would respond successfully to eradication with no recurrence of symptoms, is sufficiently high to ensure that the expected total cost per patient is lower than it would be to maintain them on therapy with no investigations for the remainder of their life. Not only is the suggestion that testing for *H. pylori* may be financially beneficial from the GP viewpoint, but it would seem logical to assume that most patients would prefer to have the opportunity for successful treatment of their symptoms without long-term medication. Frequent ad hoc comments from patients expressed a feeling of 'well-being' following successful eradication of the infection. Of this study group, 52% of patients were identified as *H. pylori*-positive, successfully treated first time and did not experience any recurrence of symptoms within a six-month period. Utilising the skills and time of a pharmacist to counsel and provide health promotion may have contributed to good patient compliance and may have influenced this outcome. Further long-term follow-up of these patients will be required before the longer-term success or otherwise can be determined.

Sixty-two percent of patients without a confirmed diagnosis remained symptom-free six months post-*H. pylori* eradication. The total expected cost per patient for maintenance therapy over remaining life expectancy is greater than testing for *H. pylori* and treating accordingly.

While the number of patients in this group was small, the results suggest that further research in this area is needed, not only from a patient viewpoint but also bearing in mind the financial implications.

Patients with dyspepsia presenting for the first time

There is concern that too frequent use of eradication therapy will result in antibiotic resistance. Antibiotic resistance and its association with over-use of antibiotics has recently been given a high profile (SMAC, 1998). However, many patients presenting to their general practitioner with dyspepsia have symptoms suggestive of peptic ulcer. Where a course of antacid fails, current accepted options would be either to refer for endoscopy or to treat with a course of an ulcer-healing agent. Except in patients with 'alarm' symptoms, where early endoscopy to exclude cancer is necessary, most of these patients would be treated in primary care with a course of an ulcer-healing agent. Unfortunately, this often leads to long-term repeat prescriptions, at least intermittently. Furthermore, many of these patients will be treated with a H$_2$RA or PPI, which may be inappropriate if the patient is *H. pylori*-positive. The alternative approach of testing and eradicating is not only a more cost-effective approach but 95% of the new presentations required no further treatment at least six months after receiving a course of eradication therapy. We, therefore, considered that the benefits gained from this approach outweighed any potential risk of antibiotic resistance.

It would appear from this small study that clinical benefit and direct financial savings can be achieved if, in addition to patients with a diagnosis of duodenal ulcer or gastric ulcer, all patients on long-term H$_2$RA or PPI therapy are treated for *H. pylori* infection. However, decision analysis was based on a small patient sample, from one general practice, and required input from previous literature to develop it. Larger studies in primary care with long-term follow-up post eradication will need to be undertaken to confirm the potential benefits of application on a wider scale.

Although the majority of patients with dyspepsia are managed by their general practitioners, most of the research has taken place in selected hospital populations and thus most of the literature on *H. pylori* originates from secondary care. This may have introduced bias in the guidelines produced nationally (SIGN, 1996). Until sufficient research is based in general practice, a lower level of evidence might be applied to general practitioner views, provided this is backed by experience and common sense.

Conclusion

Treatment of upper gastrointestinal disease represents a significant workload and has major financial implications in primary care. A system-based approach to disease management ensures that patients receive the best available treatment according to current evidence-based medicine, delivered effectively and efficiently. Only two professional groups within primary care have the skills to arrange systems of care: general practitioners and pharmacists. The general practitioner partners in this study believed that pharmacists are more able to dedicate time to disease management clinics, since patients seeing a doctor expect other problems they may have to be dealt with at the same time. Delegation of responsibility for some of the more routine patient care in this way should reduce some of the burden currently placed on general practitioners. It will also allow doctors to take on more specialised services in primary care, reducing the need for hospitals to deal with minor problems, which can be managed in the general practice surgery. Once a medical diagnosis has been made, pharmacists can use their knowledge to select an appropriate medicine for the individual patient, based on the diagnosis, concurrent medical problems and other medicines being prescribed. Tailoring of doses, counselling to prepare patients for possible side effects and how to manage them and monitoring for the occurrence of long-term adverse effects can also be realised. This can be achieved through structured review of patients and adherence to systems to manage new presentations and without conflict of interest between general practitioners and pharmacists, with doctors retaining ultimate responsibility for their patients. In the example reported in this chapter, the result of this strategy is that expenditure on ulcer-healing medicines is reducing at practice level, despite increases throughout the UK.

Pharmacists are currently one of the most under-utilised healthcare professionals in the NHS. Their unique skills are beginning to receive recognition by general practitioners (Dunbar 1997; Wells 1997; Wells 1998). Furthermore, NHS healthcare planners recognise the need for a rational approach to the use of medicines to secure optimal patient care within finite resources. The problem of drug-related morbidity and mortality requires attention and pharmaceutical care could potentially make a significant contribution to resolving it. The concept of disease management clinics combining medication review and pharmaceutical care with the use of guidelines, provides many new opportunities for pharmacists to expand and develop their role, using their professional skills to secure a more positive and challenging future. This model could be adapted for other disease states where medication plays an important role in the treatment and may be a practical approach to the local implementation of evidence-based guidelines. However, pharmacists' contribution to healthcare and cost-effectiveness in the future is unlikely to be achieved within traditional doctor-centred practices. Quality improvement programmes based on total quality management principles have been shown to produce beneficial changes in service delivery and team working in most general practices (Lawrence and Packwood, 1996). This was undoubtedly one of the essential components that contributed to a successful outcome for patients in this study. The integration of pharmacists into primary healthcare teams can encourage a systematic approach to the organisation of disease management for patients. Pharmacists can also ensure provision of high and assured quality care with both patient and general practitioner appreciation. Widespread implementation offers an exciting future for the pharmacist.

Acknowledgements

I would like to thank all the staff and patients at Downfield Surgery, Dundee, for their part in this study. I would also like to thank Dr James Dunbar, Medical Director, Borders Primary Care Trust, Professor John Cromarty, Acute Trust Chief Pharmacist, Highland, John Hamley, Primary Care Trust Chief Pharmacist, Tayside, Professor Mo Malek and Dr Anne-Marie McIntyre, Pharmaco-economic Research Centre, University of St Andrews, for their specific input.

The study was funded by a pharmacy practice research grant from the Scottish Office Home and Health Department.

References

Anonymous (1997). Helicobacter pylori testing kits. *Drug Ther Bull* 35: 23–24.

Axon A T R (1993). Helicobacter pylori infection. *J Antimicrob Chemother* 32(Suppl A): 61–8.

Barnes J (1995). Helicobacter pylori eradication up to date. *Practitioner* 239: 67–68.

Briggs A H, Sculpher M J, Logan R P H, *et al.* (1996). Cost effectiveness of screening for and eradication of Helicobacter pylori in management of dyspeptic patients under 45 years of age. *BMJ* 312: 1321–25.

Brown D J, Helling D K, Jones M E (1979). Evaluation of clinical pharmacists consultations in a family practice office. *Am J Hosp Pharm* 36: 912–15.

Cipolle R J, Strand L M, Morley P C (1998). *Pharmaceutical Care Practice.* New York: McGraw-Hill.

Coast-Senior E A, Kroner B A, Kelley C L, *et al.* (1998). Management of patients with type 2 diabetes by pharmacists in primary care clinics. *Ann Pharmacother* 32(6): 636–41.

Craig A M, Malek M, Davey P, *et al.* (1996). Economic evaluation with decision analysis: is it useful for medical decision making? The case of acute uncomplicated cystitis in women. *Br J Med Economics* 10: 275–90.

De Boer W A, van Etten R J, Scahde R W, *et al.* (1997). One-day intensified lansoprazole-quadruple therapy for cure of Helicobacter pylori infection. *Aliment Pharmacol Ther* 11: 109–12.

Dunbar J A, Macgregor S H (1997). The challenge of managed care and disease management for primary care in the UK. *J Managed Care* 1: 68–72.

Furmega E M (1993). Pharmacist management of a hyperlipideamia clinic. *Am J Hosp Pharm* 50(1): 91–5.

Goudie B M, McKenzie P E, Cupriano J, *et al.* (1996). Repeat prescribing of ulcer healing drugs in general practice – prevalence and underlying diagnosis. *Aliment Pharmacol Ther* 10: 147–50.

Grol R (1992). Implementing guidelines in general practice care. *Quality in Health Care* 1: 184–91.

Hallissey M T, Allum W H, Jewkes A J, *et al.* (1990). Early detection of gastric cancer. *BMJ* 301: 513–15.

Hart L L, Evans D C, Welker R G, *et al.* (1979). The Clinical Pharmacist on a multi-disciplinary primary health care team. *Drug Intell Clin Pharm* 13: 414–19.

Hawkey C J (1994). Eradication of Helicobacter pylori should be pivotal in managing peptic ulceration: eradication largely prevents relapse. *BMJ* 309: 1570–72.

Haxby D G, Weart C W, Goodman B W (1988). Family Practice physician's perceptions of the usefullness of drug therapy recommendations from clinical pharmacists. *Am J Hosp Pharm* 45: 824–27.

Hepler C D, Strand L M (1990). Opportunities and responsibilities in pharmaceutical care. *Am J Hosp Pharm* 47: 533–43.

Kosunen T U, Seppala K, Sarna S, *et al.* (1992). Diagnostic value of decreasing IgG, IgA and IgM antibody titres after eradication of Helicobacter pylori. *Lancet* 339: 893–95.

Kung N N, Sung J J, Yuen N W, *et al.* (1997). Anti Helicobacter pylori treatment in bleeding ulcer: randomised controlled trial comparing 2 day versus 7 day bismuth quadruple therapy. *Am J Gastroenterol* 92: 438–41.

Lawrence M, Packwood T (1996). Adapting total quality management for general practice: evaluation of a programme. *Quality in Health Care* 5(3): 151–58.

Lima H A (1998). Disease management in the alternate-site health care setting. *Am J Health Syst Pharm* 55(5): 471–76.

Macgregor S H, Hamley J G, Dunbar J A, *et al.* (1996). Evaluation of a primary care anticoagulant clinic run by a pharmacist. *BMJ* 312: 560.

McIntyre A M, Macgregor S, Malek M, *et al.* (1997). New patients presenting to their GP with dyspepsia: does Helicobacter pylori eradication minimise the cost of managing these patients? *Int J Clin Pract* 51(5): 276–81.

MEL (1993). *Scottish Home and Health Department accountability review: priorities and planning guidelines for 1994/95.* 155.

NIH Consensus Development Panel (1994). Helicobacter pylori in peptic ulcer disease. *J Am Med Assoc* 272: 66–9.

Perry P J, Hurley S C (1975). Activities of the clinical pharmacist practising in the office of a family practitioner. *Drug Intell Clin Pharm.* 9: 129–33.

SIGN (Scottish Intercollegiate Guideline Network) (1996). *Helicobacter pylori: eradication therapy in dyspeptic disease.*

SMAC (Standing Medical Advisory Committee) (1998). *The path of least resistance.* Department of Health.

Tytgat G N J (1994). Review article: treatments that impact favourably upon the eradication of Helicobacter pylori and ulcer recurrence. *Aliment Pharmacol Ther* 8: 359–68.

Wells D (1997). Pharmacists are key members of primary health care teams. *BMJ* 314: 1486.

Wells D (1998). Having a practice pharmacist can reduce prescribing costs. *BMJ* 317: 473.

Wensing M, Van der Weijden T, Grol R (1998). Implementing guidelines and innovations in general practice: which interventions are effective? *Br J Gen Pract* 48: 991–97.

7

Hospital at home

Sharon Williams

Introduction

The term 'hospital at home' (HAH) relates to the provision of hospital-level treatment to patients who continue to live in their own home. For the purposes of this chapter, 'hospital at home' refers to those models of care that involve home-stay patients receiving some form of intravenous (IV) therapy that may or may not be self-administered. These models are known by terms such as 'non-inpatient IV care' (NIPIV), 'home infusion therapy programmes' (HITP), 'out-patient intravenous antimicrobial therapy' (OPAT), or 'alternate site infusion'.

The concepts of 'hospital at home' care originated in North America early in the 1970s, driven by the desire to reduce the costs of healthcare to patients (Catania, 1994). One of the first indications for which HAH care was used, was chronic bronchopulmonary infection associated with cystic fibrosis (Rucker and Harrison, 1974). These workers found that almost 70% of hospitalisations could be avoided and this was associated with the benefits of fiscal savings in medical costs, lack of disruption of family routine and, in some cases, continuation of schooling and employment. Since this initial report, many studies have demonstrated the efficacy, relative safety, reduction in cross-infection and cost savings associated with this type of service (Stiver *et al.*, 1978; Stiver *et al.*, 1982; Rehm and Weinstein, 1983; Kind, 1985; Sharp, 1986; Chamberlain *et al.*, 1988; Glick, 1991; Wiernikowski, 1991; Bernstein, 1991; Scully, 1992; Thickson, 1993; Rubinstein, 1993). The essential criteria which underpin successful HAH services are: careful selection of motivated patients; suitable home circumstances; multidisciplinary input; and good communication channels between all team members (Stiver *et al.*, 1982; Rehm and Weinstein, 1983; Kind, 1985; Sharp, 1986; Simmons *et al.*, 1990; Rich, 1994; Tice, 1996; Watters, 1997).

Poretz *et al.* (1984) performed a cost benefit analysis of home IV therapy, in which all quantifiable benefits, e.g. increased productivity or return to work or school, were measured. They determined a mean total benefit of $6588 per patient, and a mean total cost of $1768 per patient. The conclusion of the study was 'for all parties concerned, the benefits of outpatient IV therapy versus hospital IV therapy far outweigh the costs'. A HAH infrastructure (Milkovich, 1995) is now well established in North America to cover indications such as: oncology chemotherapy (DeMoss, 1980; Jayabose et al., 1992; McCorkle, 1994; Shane, 1996); renal dialysis (NAIT, 1993); total parenteral nutrition (Jeejeebhoy, 1973; Shils, 1975; Heizer, 1977; Raehl, 1993; Hatwig, 1996); pain (Raehl, 1993); a myriad of infections (Sharp, 1986; Chamberlain et al., 1988; Glick, 1991; Wiernikowski, 1991; Bernstein, 1991; Scully, 1992; Rubinstein, 1993; Williams, 1995; Hatwig, 1996); haemophilia (Raehl, 1993); severe heart failure (Dies, 1986; Collins, 1990; Phillips, 1992; Miller, 1994; Marius-Nunez et al., 1996); and even blood infusions (Benson, 1997). Regardless of how the programme is organised, the service appears to be well accepted by patients and third party payers provided it is organised in an efficient manner. However, worry and uncertainty can be an intangible cost to the patient and carers when a programme lacks organisation and a regular point of contact. This was amply demonstrated by Nolet (1989), who showed how lack of information and disorganisation of a HAH programme can lead to patient lack of confidence in the system and the subsequent desire to be treated in

Table 7.1 Comparison of the costs of IV HAH care

	Hospital	*HAH*
Direct costs	Hospitalisation	–
	Drugs	Drugs
	Consumables	Consumables
	Staff time	Patient/carer time
		IV technique training
Indirect costs	Loss of income	Commuting costs for clinic
	Interruption of education	follow-up
	Family commuting costs	
Intangible costs	Dependence	Worry and uncertainty
	Depression	
	Confinement	
	Separation from family	

hospital. Table 7.1 compares and contrasts the various costs of HAH care with in-hospital care.

Quality assurance

Since the early 1970s the number of people receiving HAH services has grown exponentially. In 1993, Tice estimated that approximately 250 000 North American patients were being treated per annum. This growth stimulated the Joint Commission on Accreditation of Healthcare Organisations (JCAHO) to develop accreditation standards for provider organisations (Malloy, 1990). Quality assurance of home IV services must incorporate standards for the structure through which care is given, the process of selecting, assessing, training and treating patients and indicators of clinical outcome. An organisation, which earns accreditation by operating to JCAHO standards, demonstrates to the consumer and payer a commitment to providing the highest level of quality care and service. Other information on which to base practice is given by Home Infusion Therapy Indicators (Kunkel, 1993) and Quality Indicator Groups System for intravenous infusion therapy (Shaughnessy, 1989). Guidelines on the pharmacist's role in home care have also been provided by the regulatory body of American hospital pharmacists (ASHP, 1993). This document details all aspects of a pharmacist's responsibility in home healthcare such as initial patient assessment, patient education, training and counselling, development of pharmaceutical care plans, patient clinical monitoring, communication pathways etc.

A new jargon is evolving in North America to describe the potential problems of home IV therapy. For example, the adjective nosohusial (home-acquired) has been suggested as a parallel term to nosocomial (hospital-acquired) in the descriptions of infections (Graham, 1993). Guidelines for control of infection at home need to be incorporated into quality assurance models (Simmons, 1990).

Safety and 'acceptable risk'

Given the predisposition that North Americans have for litigation it would be reasonable to assume that a vast literature concerning safety and legal issues would exist, but this does not appear to be the case. Safety aspects are referred to in the literature but it is somewhat fragmentary. An explanation for this may be that HAH care developed in order to reduce the costs of treatment to patients. Apparently, North American patients have implicitly accepted the risk of an adverse event occurring at home for the benefits of convenience and lower care costs. From available information, adverse reaction frequency appears to be no greater than that occurring in hospital and this has come to be considered an 'acceptable risk'. In one of the first reports of HAH care, Rucker et al. (1974) stated that no major complications were noted, although mild phlebitis necessitating IV-line resiting was required after seven to eight days in some patients. Stiver et al. (1978) concluded that side effects were no different from those in in-hospital treated patients and that there was actually a decreased prevalence of phlebitis in patients treated at home. In a review of North American HAH literature, Balinsky et al. (1989) concluded 'there currently exists sufficient data to support both the safety and clinical effectiveness of outpatient parenteral antibiotic therapy'. This conclusion has continued to be endorsed by others (Bernstein, 1991; Grizzard, 1991; Graham, 1991; Williams, 1993).

However, the quantification of 'acceptable risk' from the existing literature is somewhat nebulous. Cote et al. (1989) carried out a 12-year review of the Manitoba home IV antibiotic programme, in which there had been 748 admissions to the programme equating to 15 366 patient days. During this time, phlebitis was occurring at a rate of 14.7% and there had been seven penicillin-induced allergic reactions, one reaction was severe leading to respiratory failure requiring resuscitation. Despite this, the overall conclusion was that the programme was safe and effective. Implicit in this conclusion, therefore, is that phlebitis occurring at 14.7% and one respiratory failure for 748 admissions constitutes 'acceptable risk' to this particular healthcare provider and associated consumers. Adverse event rates vary between individual drugs and so, therefore, will the 'acceptable' risk (New et al., 1991; Tice, 1991; Morales, 1994).

Role of the pharmacist in North American HAH care

The pharmacist is an integral member of North American HAH programmes (Stiver et al., 1982; Rehm and Weinstein, 1983; Kind, 1985; Sharp, 1986; Raehl et al., 1993; Tice, 1996). The three main providers of these programmes are hospitals, home infusion companies and primary care physician offices. Regardless of where the home programme is based, a quality programme requires close communication between physician, nurse and pharmacist to ensure that the patient is being managed as the physician intended (Simmons et al., 1990; Watters, 1997). The specific responsibilities of pharmacists may vary depending on whether they are office-based or work for a home infusion company or hospital, but several responsibilities are universal. In addition to the traditional role of the pharmacist in drug compounding, dispensing and supply, the pharmacist is responsible for advising on selection of appropriate drug, technology and devices to be used for administration in the home. The pharmacists are frequently involved in the initial assessment of a patient prior to enrolment onto a HAH programme. Other duties include education and instruction of patients and care-givers about the use, administration and storage of medications, in addition to being a source of professional education and drug information for other members of the healthcare team. The pharmacist is involved in assessing the patient's goals for drug therapy; monitoring the patient for possible development of drug-related problems (e.g. drug interactions, toxicity); and keeping abreast of the patient's progress. Lastly, the pharmacist assists the patient with waste management, particularly the disposal of hazardous and contaminated waste products.

HAH care in the UK

Although the largest number of publications relating to IV HAH care services are North American in origin, other countries do have similar established services (Charles, 1990; Kawaguchi *et al.*, 1994; Monalto *et al.*, 1998; Sindone *et al.*, 1998; Anonymous, 1998). By comparison, provision of IV HAH care in the UK is not as structured and has developed at a much slower pace. Provision, however, is more widely disseminated than is first suggested by the paucity of UK literature. Reports of HAH care have generally been provided by individual units within some hospitals and limited to a few indications, such as: cystic fibrosis with recurrent infection (Gilbert *et al.*, 1988; Agnew, 1997); oncology patients (Sewell *et al.*, 1987; Rolston, 1995; Williams, 1998); long-term parenteral nutritional support (Malone, 1994; Elia, 1995; Richards *et al.*, 1997); pain management (Dover, 1988); and AIDS (Kayley *et al.*, 1996; Agnew, 1997; Wiselka *et al.*, 1997). Secondary care institutions are not isolated in their provision; it is known that a Dundee community pharmacist (Brown, 1998) has provided long-term HAH parenteral nutritional support services and is currently involved in the development of an IV pain management programme for terminally ill patients. On a slightly larger scale, the commercial company SunScript has been providing community parenteral nutritional support services since 1995 (Anonymous, 1998). Demand for IV HAH provision is developing as evidenced by a recent 'invitation to tender' notice by the Royal Brompton and Harefield NHS Trust, London.

A reason for the slow maturation of HAH care in the UK may relate to the unchallenged culture and belief that IV therapy necessitates hospitalisation. The force driving the development of this care in North America was a desire to reduce the costs of treatment to patients (Rucker and Harrison, 1974; Stiver *et al.*, 1982; Poretz *et al.*, 1982; Rehm and Weinstein, 1983; Sharp, 1986; Chamberlain *et al.*, 1988). Contrary to this, the driving force for the provision of HAH care in the UK has been quality of life factors (Gilbert and Littlewood, 1988; BPA Working Party on Cystic Fibrosis, 1988).

The research question

Given the wide-ranging reports of cost-effectiveness of North American IV HAH care, its wider application in the UK deserves further investigation. Direct extrapolation of cost-effectiveness is problematic due to the differing ways each healthcare infrastructure is financed.

A study designed to examine the logistics, costs and benefits of IV HAH for acute infection was undertaken in the Infectious Diseases Unit (IDU) of Dundee Acute Hospitals NHS Trust, Tayside, during 1994. The research question was to determine whether home IV antibiotic treatment for acute infections was feasible in the UK. Three perspectives were considered, those of the patients, the initial secondary care provider and other healthcare professionals who could become involved in the provision of this service. The study team was multidisciplinary, comprising pharmacy, medical and nursing staff.

The objectives of this study were:

- To determine which patients are suitable for IV antibiotic HAH care.
- To determine how practical provision of this service would be in Tayside.
- To quantify the costs and benefits of IV HAH treatment versus in-patient IV treatment.
- To evaluate the perceptions of both study patients and Tayside General Practitioners (GPs) of this type of service.

The study

The study design

The study design was centred around discharging patients with infection requiring IV antibiotic therapy to their home as soon as they were clinically stable. The study incorporated two arms: IV antibiotic administration as a hospital outpatient and patient/carer IV antibiotic administration in the home environment. The antibiotics used in the study were ceftriaxone and teicoplanin; they were chosen for their spectrum of activity and requirements of once-daily administration. It was intended that equal numbers of patients would be randomised to receive either one or other of the antibiotics; this was pragmatically moderated to take into account identified pathogen sensitivity. Clinical responsibility was maintained by the hospital for patients at all times during the study period. Domiciliary visits were not undertaken. Ethics approval was sought and granted.

Patients and methods

From January to November 1994 all patients admitted to the IDU of Dundee Acute Hospitals were considered for IV HAH care. The unit was the regional unit for treating adults with infection, serving a population of approximately 400 000. The unit comprised 54 beds, 28 devoted to orthopaedic patients with an infective complication, the remainder being assigned to patients with any other infection. The majority of admissions were direct referrals from primary care general practitioners but a significant number of referrals were from other units within the trust.

Patient selection

Patients receiving IV antibiotics for 24 hours were evaluated by a senior member of the study team to determine whether the patient was a prospective candidate for the HAH programme. This required that the patient be medically stable, was expected to require the IV route of administration for at least five days and had an infection amenable to either ceftriaxone or teicoplanin. On meeting these criteria, the patient was then socially assessed by the study pharmacist through a personal, interactive, semi-structured interview. Encouragement was given to the patient to have a family member or friend present at the interview. Several hours prior to interview, an information sheet, which explained the background and reasons for the study, was given to each of the patients so that they could discuss it with their family/friends if they so desired; it also gave patients the opportunity to formulate any questions. At interview all aspects of the study were explained and the opportunity was given for the patient to ask as many questions as they wished. Each interview lasted approximately 30 minutes. The social assessment included fully informing the patient of all aspects of the study, determining that the patient was motivated and willing to participate and that home circumstances were supportive for this form of therapy, for example, easy access to a telephone, and suitable drug storage facilities. Suitability of home circumstance was taken on trust and a value judgement of the patient; domiciliary visits were not undertaken. At this point written informed consent was obtained from those wishing to participate.

Organisation of treatment

Antibiotic administration as an outpatient   Patients were provided with an information sheet explaining about the antibiotic that they would receive, the expected duration of treatment and the need to return to the ward daily to receive treatment. The information sheet also explained about possible side effects and complications of treatment such as phlebitis. Outpatient treatment was administered daily on one of the wards, mostly by a member of the medical staff. During this visit the patient's IV access and clinical progress was also briefly assessed. To provide support for patients at home a 24-hour staff contact cascade system was provided.

Patient/carer IV antibiotic administration in the home environment   As with the outpatient arm of the study, patients were provided with an information sheet explaining about the antibiotic they would receive and the expected duration of treatment.

Patients or their carers were trained by the study pharmacist to prepare and administer the injections on the ward and observed to ensure correct practice on two occasions. In addition to all required supplies, patients were provided with an instruction booklet to take home. The booklet listed the supplies required, provided a quick reference reminder followed by detailed instructions for preparation and administration, outlined possible complications and provided a 24-hour staff contact cascade system. Patients were asked to return to the ward twice weekly to review IV access and clinical condition.

Patient transport   At the point of discharge to home, transport arrangements and review dates and times for return to the hospital were confirmed. Transport arrangements included a private facility (taxi) or reimbursement of travel costs, whichever the patient preferred. The time arranged for attendance at the hospital was that which was convenient to the patient. This allowed those patients returning to work to attend either before or after the working day.

Clinical responsibility   Although clinical responsibility was maintained by the hospital for the patient during the study period, each patient's general practitioner was contacted on the day of discharge to their home to give notification that the patient would be in the community with an IV access in situ. The general practitioners and members of the community nursing team were not asked to be directly involved in the study. Furthermore, no hospital-based member of the team visited the patient at home but advice and support was available at all times.

Fiscal evaluation   Detailed financial accounting of all drugs and consumables used was recorded for each patient, including those consumables used in providing an IV access. Note was also taken of the amount of staff time required for patient continuing care. Total transportation costs, or distance travelled, were recorded for each patient. In order to create a comparable costing for hospital-based treatments, two Infectious Diseases (ID) consultants independently made an estimate, based on the clinical history, of what therapy these patients would have reasonably received had they remained in hospital. Treatment was defined according to the written guidelines in the IDU. These guidelines specify the drug, dose, route of administration and duration of treatment. The consultants also estimated the length of patient stay. This allowed all direct costs (drugs, consumables, staff time) of study treatment to be compared and contrasted with the standard direct inpatient treatment costs had the patient remained as an inpatient.

General practitioner attitude to IV HAH care   A telephone survey of all Tayside GP teams was carried out to determine their attitude to the provision of a HAH service. This was achieved by initially contacting each practice by letter, briefly explaining the reasons for and the purpose of an IV HAH service and providing a copy of the questions to be explored at interview. Contact was then made by telephone to arrange a suitable time to carry out the interview. Although only one partner per practice was interviewed, it was assumed (as requested) that the views expressed were a consensus of all the partners in the practice.

Patient preferences   Patients' perceptions of the benefits and drawbacks of IV HAH care were assessed via a semi-structured interview prior to treatment and a self-completed open-ended questionnaire after treatment.

Additional information was obtained from a focus group meeting of study patients which was conducted by staff who had not previously met the patients.

Results

Study population characteristics

During an 11-month period, 1057 patients were admitted to the IDU. Only those patients prescribed antibiotics (559) were eligible for the study. More than 50% of these patients (304/559) received antibiotics by the oral route, leaving a sub-group of 255 (24% of original admission population) patients from which to recruit. From this sub-group 24 patients met the initial criteria and were socially suitable for entry into the study. Table 7.2 shows the reasons for non-recruitment of the other 231 patients, the main reasons were short-term need of parenteral antibiotics and medical instability.

However, social circumstances that may have been surmountable with greater community support were a factor in 25 patients, for example, one young mother of five children suffering from an orbital cellulitis felt she would have 'no peace' if she returned home. A further two patients were recruited to the study from the ID outpatients clinic and another three were referred to the study from other units in the hospital, giving a final total of 29 study patients. The reasons for IV treatment of the study patients in preference to oral therapy are given in Table 7.3.

Recruited patient age ranged from 17–75 years and the length of treatment ranged from [a]1–88 days. The longest length of treatment for the home arm was 69 days and 88 days for the outpatient arm. The major indication for HAH treatment was skin and soft tissue infection, accounting for over 50% of patients, with the remainder of patients

Table 7.2 Reasons for non-recruitment of patients receiving IV antibiotics onto the HAH study

Reasons for non-recruitment	No of patients
Short-term IV antibiotics (<5 days)	186
Medically unstable	20
Socially not suitable (e.g. history of depression, too infirm, etc.)	19
Other (e.g. too far to travel, study antibiotic unsuitable)	6

[a]One patient discontinued antibiotic treatment after one day because of a changed diagnosis.

Table 7.3 Reasons for IV route of administration versus oral route

•   Failure of oral therapy.
•   Immunocompromised.
•   Serious infection – need to ensure high serum levels.
•   Underlying pathology, e.g. diabetes.
•   Ramadan.

having a variety of infections. A larger proportion of patients were treated as outpatients, (19, versus 10 patients in the home arm).

Costs of treatment

The average cost per HAH study patient was £665, compared with the predicted average cost of £427 for inpatient treatment. This indicates average additional costs of £261 per patient for HAH therapy. However, exclusion of orthopaedic patients reduced the additional cost of HAH care to £62. Orthopaedic infections are associated with particularly high treatment costs because of their chronicity and therefore duration of treatment required. The average cost of treating an orthopaedic patient was £2548 in the HAH programme, compared to £1523 had the patient been treated as an inpatient, giving an additional cost of £1025 for the HAH programme.

Overall HAH costs for the 29 study patients exceeded the hypothetical inpatient treatment costs by just over £6600. This was primarily brought about by the difference in drug acquisition costs. The acquisition costs of the drugs used in the study exceeded those that would have been used in the hospital by 70% (£17 219 compared with £10 030), to a small extent this was offset by the HAH consumable costs being lower than those for inpatient treatment (£464 compared with £1369). For a fuller discussion of these costs and sub-group cost effectiveness see Parker *et al.* (1998).

Impact of the HAH programme on utilisation of hospital bed days

The total number of bed days saved by the 29 patients on the programme totalled 532, representing an average of 18 bed days per patient. However, this figure is skewed by five orthopaedic patients who accounted for almost 60% (316) of these bed days. The average number of bed days saved per non-orthopaedic patient was 9 days, with a median of 5.5 days, which is in stark comparison to the average of 63 days and median of 62 days for an orthopaedic patient.

Total bed day capacity of the ID unit was 19,710 for 1994. Thus, the 532 days saved by those patients on the programme represented only 2.7%. Capacity utilisation for the ID unit was assumed to be around 45%, based on the preceding three years average, and so the 532 bed days saved represented 4% of 1994 expected actual bed day consumption.

At the time of this feasibility study the 'hotel cost' per bed day in the ID Unit was calculated to be £313 (Scottish Health Service Costs, 1994). It could be argued, therefore, that £166 516 (532 × £313) had been saved; however, unless the savings could be made tangible by reducing fixed costs, this argument would be flawed. Considerable rationalisation of the ID service has taken place and in 1996 the number of inpatient beds was reduced to 35; 22 on the Kings Cross site and 12 in a new Orthopaedic Infection Unit at Dundee Royal Infirmary (DRI). Nonetheless, at the level of 29 patients per year, HAH therapy would still have a minimal effect, even on this reduced bed capacity. Following Trust reorganisation in the late 90s, DRI has closed, with all beds transferring to Ninewells Hospital.

Transportation costs

Of the 29 patients, 14 requested or required the taxi transportation proffered, the remainder chose to use their own transport. Although the patients using their own transport had the opportunity for travel reimbursement to the hospital no patient opted for this. Where taxi transportation was provided the average cost was £114 per patient. However, four were orthopaedic patients who required transportation for 28 days or longer, their average cost was £266 per patient, giving an average cost of £53 per patient for the remaining group.

Perspectives of patients who received HAH treatment

Table 7.4 summarises the anticipated benefits that patients believed HAH IV treatment would bring.

The most frequently cited advantage was the freedom afforded of being at home. During the screening process patients were also asked whether they or their relatives had concerns of any nature regarding HAH care. Of the 29 patients, 26 had no personal concerns whatsoever, three had concerns which were of a low-level nature in that the concerns did not deter the patient from participating in the programme. Sixteen

Table 7.4 Patient benefits of IV HAH treatment – anticipated before treatment (n = 29, 60 responses) and experienced during treatment (n = 26, 60 responses)

Benefit	% anticipated	% experienced
Freedom of being at home, e.g. cook, shopping, sleep in own bed, etc.	79	85
Less stressful	38	19
Can return to work/deal with personal matters	31	62
Less family disruption	31	38
Increased social contact	21	27

patients had chosen to discuss entry into the programme with a close relative or friend and 13 had not. Of the 16 patients who did discuss the HAH programme with a relative or friend, four relatives expressed concerns. The nature of the concerns expressed both by patients and relatives are given in Table 7.5.

Of the 29 study patients, 26 completed the 'end of study' questionnaires, one patient did not return the questionnaire, one patient died and the remaining patient was removed from the study after their initial diagnosis was changed after one day of HAH care. The vast majority of patients, 92% (24), said they would repeat this form of therapy again; The two patients (8%) who said they wouldn't, considered that they would have had more rest had they remained in hospital. Five patients (19%) thought that HAH had caused them 'out of pocket' expenses but qualified this by stating that this was of their own choice. The perceived advantages of the patients prior to participating in the study were corroborated by the actual advantages experienced (Table 7.4).

Table 7.5 Concerns about IV HAH treatment expressed by patients and relatives

Nature of patient-expressed concern	Nature of relative-expressed concern
• Feels safer in hospital but self-rationalised that this is because this form of treatment is a new idea	• Mother (×2) concerned that the level of care given by the HAH programme might not be the same as in hospital
• Could envisage difficulties arranging for children to be cared for	• Wife thought that better treatment would be given in hospital
• Didn't like the idea of having an IV access in situ at home	• Wife needed reassurance that it was OK for her husband to go home with an infection

Nine patients treated by the HAH programme between January and August 1994 participated in a focus group discussion, all stated they would repeat this form of therapy and felt the treatment at home improved their quality of life. Table 7.6 summarises the key points raised by this group.

GP perspective of HAH treatment

A response to the summary letter circulated to 61 general practitioner practices representing 295 individual general practitioners was obtained from 41 practices (representing 125 general practitioners). Not all practices responded to all questions. When asked about the advantages/disadvantages of a HAH service to both themselves and to their patients, a large proportion (71%) anticipated no advantage to themselves and a substantial number anticipated disadvantage (46%) in the form of an increased workload. When considering the patients' potential benefits of a HAH service, the majority of general practitioners thought that the patients would gain from getting home more quickly and being in their own environment. The disadvantages to the patients discussed by the general practitioners varied widely but all centred around the lack of experience of this type of therapy. Various options for how HAH care could be organised was presented to the general practitioners The majority felt they could only support HAH care when both funding and responsibility remained within the secondary care sector. For further information see Parker *et al.* (1998).

Table 7.6 Summary of key points from patient focus discussion group

• Reaction to IV HAH care was favourable, the principal benefits being the ability to recuperate at home and to go back to work if so desired.
• The organization of the service was effective.
• The service was perceived positively by all respondents.
• GPs had limited awareness and knowledge of the service.
• No one said that the family/carers had expressed a concern about the treatment.
• Several ways were suggested to make the service even better. These included: – a specific location for the service;   – appointments;   – a single named contact person;   – creating greater awareness amongst GPs.

Safety of HAH care

Eight patients (27.6% of study population) reported a medical-related problem associated with their HAH care. The type of problem expressed by six patients was considered to be of a minor nature, related to either the speed of injection or to the discomfort (phlebitis) caused by the IV access. The problem experienced by the remaining two patients (6.9% of study population) was of a more serious nature. Both these patients displayed a hypersensitivity type reaction whilst receiving antibiotic treatment as outpatients. The first reaction followed administration of a second dose of teicoplanin which was being used to treat a right leg cellulitis. The antibiotic had been administered within the hospital, with the patient then returning home. The onset of symptoms (rigours, global piloerection, dry mouth, chest tightness and shortness of breath) occurred some 60 minutes post-dose, the episode being of approximately 20 minutes duration. The patient contacted the hospital during the episode and although advised to return to the ward the patient declined but returned the following day. Treatment was changed to ceftriaxone, the patient continued on the programme and the infection was success-fully treated. The second reaction was experienced by a patient being treated with ceftriaxone for osteomyelitis of the right temporal bone. The reaction was first experienced some 30 days after initial antibiotic administration and took the form of a transient flushing sensation in the face and neck immediately following antibiotic administration. From this point forward the patient reported an increasing degree of transient flushing sensation on administration of ceftriaxone. An antihistamine (terfenadine, 60 mg twice daily) was administered to try to ameliorate the problem but with little success. Antibiotic administration was stopped 26 days after the first report of 'flushing'. On follow-up the patient reported that the reaction had abated. During the antibiotic treatment, this patient was also taking medication (isosorbide mono-nitrate, glyceryl trinitrate, frusemide, aspirin, amlodipine, lisinopril) for underlying pathology of ischaemic heart and peripheral vascular disease. However, given the circumstantial evidence it was felt that the 'flushing' reaction was in fact due to the ceftriaxone rather than the other chronic medication.

Discussion

The stimuli for this feasibility study were the consistent reports from the US on the cost effectiveness and patient popularity of HAH services. The experience encountered in this study reflects both similarities and dissimilarities with these reports. The similarities centred on workability, patient preference for such a service, and need for multidisciplinary input, the dissimilarities were of a fiscal nature and the reserved attitude of primary care physicians to their involvement in the provision of this type of service.

As in the US, the study used a multidisciplinary healthcare team and successfully demonstrated that it is logistically feasible to select and treat patients with varied acute infection in the non-inpatient setting. However, the number of patients selected over the 11-month period was relatively small, due in the main to the selection procedure, which required that patients were perceived to require antibiotics for five or more days. Seventy three percent (186/255) of patients in the IDU receiving IV antibiotics did so for less than five days. Therefore, the procedural criteria accounted for the low recruitment rate rather than medical instability which may have been expected to be more problematic, i.e. less than 10% of patients (20/255) were unsuitable for reasons of medical instability. It is entirely possible that the recruitment rate could have been substantially higher.

A surprising aspect from the patient social assessment interviews was that, although IV HAH therapy was an entirely new concept, very few patients or relatives had concerns about participating in the programme. At the end of treatment, patients expressed a consistent, distinct preference for this form of therapy when compared to the alternative of hospital inpatient care, and this was independent of the length of time a patient spent in the programme. One of the reasons for this may be that a sense of control is returned to the patient. Most problems experienced by patients were of a minor nature and neither deterred the patient from continuing on the programme nor from expressing their intention that they would readily participate again. Poretz (1993) reported that adverse drug reactions occur no more often in the HAH setting than in the hospital setting and that the incidence of phlebitis is actually lower than in the hospital. The issue of safety of HAH care was raised in this feasibility study by two patients (6.9%) experiencing an adverse event which was of a serious nature. The issue is that if an adverse event occurs within the confines of a hospital there are trained personnel on hand to deal with the problem. This security does not exist for patients in the home setting. If IV HAH care is to become as widely acceptable in the UK as it has in North America, then it will have to be considered safe by those using it. The notion of what constitutes 'acceptable risk' deserves exploration in the further development of HAH care.

There was a high correlation between perceived and actual advantages of IV HAH care expressed by the patients in this feasibility study. The most frequently cited benefit was that of having the freedom of being at home, followed by the opportunity to return to work or deal with personal matters. This desire to return to a more normal lifestyle reflects the benefits expressed by patients in the US. Furthermore, to take advantage of an earlier discharge to the home environment, study patients were prepared to incur costs to themselves by providing their own transport. Patients' perspectives should be considered in any service development, as they are the end users. The type of qualitative interview approach used in this study to elicit patients' perspectives has been found useful by others in the UK (Harries and Hill, 1994).

As previously mentioned, reports from the US consistently report cost savings associated with HAH services. The fiscal findings in this study were not as clear cut as the US reports; this is possibly due to two major differences between the UK and US. First, the reports from the US are from well-established infrastructures, designed to specifically provide HAH care. This feasibility study did not have an established infrastructure and sought to incorporate this type of service into an existing secondary care setting. Secondly, US patients and third party payers immediately realise cost savings from entry into a HAH programme as they no longer have to pay hospital 'hotel' costs. This does not happen in the UK because of the different healthcare financing system. The demand for the HAH programme generated by the feasibility study reduced bed-day consumption by a negligible 4%. It is highly unlikely, therefore, that fixed costs (staffing levels, other overheads etc.) would be decreased because of this reduction. Consequently, the potential 'hotel cost savings' of £166 516 are illusory. Decreasing fixed costs is a complex issue, as highlighted by others (Stern *et al.*, 1995). The examination of financial costs in this HAH feasibility study focused on the direct, variable treatment costs, as these could be readily identified and valid comparisons made between alternative forms of treatment. Initial inspection of these costs appeared higher than the comparative in-hospital treatment costs, therefore making HAH care appear economically unattractive. Despite this, cost-effective aspects of HAH treatment were identified by carrying out a sensitivity analysis. HAH care was found to be cost-effective provided high acquisition cost drugs were not used and treatment of long duration infection was excluded. The assumption by some workers 'that this form of therapy [i.e. HAH] would probably benefit NHS budgets' (Kayley *et al.*, 1996), and 'pharmaceutical costs are common between HAH and secondary care settings' (Knowelden *et al.*, 1991) could well be ill-founded without evidence to support the statement.

Unlike their US counterparts, the general practitioners approached in this study were somewhat reluctant to participate in the care of a patient in receipt of HAH therapy and were equally reluctant to fund this form of therapy. The consensus was that this type of service would involve an increase in workload with little benefit to themselves. This finding has been expressed by others (Curtis, 1997). Since the time of the GP survey, Government directed organisational changes have occurred, i.e. setting up of primary care groups/local healthcare co-operatives. These changes may well have changed the general practitioners' perspective.

In summary, IV antibiotic HAH care is feasible for acute infections. Patient recruitment selection criteria for this type of programme were developed, provision of a quality service was shown to be practical, and examination of the costs and benefits highlighted segments of the market (within the parameters of the study) for which this type of service initially appears to be cost-effective and not so cost-effective. Study patients expressed a high degree of preference for HAH care and were supportive for the continuation of this alternative form of therapy, even though some costs were identifiably transferred to themselves. Conversely, the majority of GPs were supportive of the idea of such a service only if there were no financial or increased workload implications. The issue of 'safety' was raised by this feasibility study, and as a result the notion of 'acceptable risk' deserves exploration in the further development of HAH care. The programme has provided a base on which further developments could expand. For example, demand for the service could be increased by including those patients who require less than five days' IV antibiotic treatment and by incorporating other conditions amenable to IV HAH therapy, such as congestive cardiac failure, peripheral vascular disease and some long-term AIDS care.

Future for pharmacy practice in IV HAH care in the UK

There is substantial evidence that an essential criterion of successful IV HAH programmes is multidisciplinary input. Published literature on IV HAH care in the UK is sparse but slowly expanding, and few studies have addressed the role of the pharmacist. This is an exciting time for service development; if pharmacists are to ensure their place as fully integrated members of the IV HAH care team they must move away from the traditional support function of dispensing and supply and use their drug knowledge and expertise to play a proactive role. Pharmacist involvement should begin with initial patient assessment of suitability for this form of care, addressing issues such as whether the patient is concordant with their other forms of drug treatment. At the discharge planning stage the pharmacist can provide advice on selection of appropriate drugs, technology and devices to be used for administration in the home and develop pharmaceutical care plans. After discharge the pharmacist will be aware of problems that may arise due to concurrent patient medication (adverse drug reactions, interactions, toxicity), can undertake therapeutic drug monitoring, can overcome the knowledge gap of patients and provide a link between hospital and home, particularly where supply of drugs (e.g. total parenteral nutrition (TPN) or cytotoxics) are provided. Pharmaceutical care augments, and is complementary to, the seamless medical and nursing care (Jennings, 1993) that these patients require. Patients must experience a high quality service, otherwise they will perceive IV HAH services as a cost-cutting exercise. Sally Allen, based at Newcastle's Royal Victoria and Associated Hospitals NHS Trust, has demonstrated how well placed 'seamless' care pharmacists are for developing and co-ordinating IV HAH programmes (Agnew, 1997).

From 1 April 1999, NHS Trusts have had statutory duties for the quality of patient care in addition to their existing financial responsibilities (Secretary of State for Health, 1997; Secretary of State for Health for Scotland, 1997). Clinical governance has been defined as the 'framework through which NHS organisations are accountable for continuously improving the quality of their services and safeguarding high standards of care by creating an environment in which excellence in clinical care will flourish' (DoH, 1998). 'Clinical governance applies to all patient services in the NHS, wherever they are provided, and to services the NHS commissions from other organisations' (NHSiS Management Executive, 1998). Given these Government directives, there can be no doubt that pharmacists have a vital role to play in establishing safe and effective pharmaceutical HAH services.

Acknowledgements

This study was sponsored by Roche Products Ltd and Hoechst Marion Roussel Ltd. We are grateful to the staff and patients for their participation in this project. This work was originally published in the Journal of Antimicrobial Therapy (Parker, 1998), and we are grateful for their permission to include it in this chapter.

References

Agnew T (1997). Deliver high tech home care. *Pharmacy in Practice.* April: 222–23.

Anonymous (1998). Importance of good communication in continuity of care. *Pharm J* 261: 548–49.

ASHP (1993). ASHP guidelines on the pharmacist's role in home care. *Am J Hosp Pharm* 50: 1940–44.

Balinsky W, Nesbitt S (1989). Cost effectiveness of outpatient parenteral antibiotics. A review of the literature. *Am J Med* 87: 301–05.

Benson K (1997). Blood transfusions in the home sweet home: How to avoid a sour outcome. Cancer Control. *JMCC* 4 (4): 364–67.

Bernstein L H (1991). An update on home intravenous antibiotic therapy. *Geriatrics* 46(6): 47–54.

BPA Working Party on cystic fibrosis (1985). Cystic Fibrosis in the United Kingdom 1977–1985: an improving picture. *BMJ* 297: 1599–602.

Brown D (1998). Personal communication. Community pharmacist, Dundee.

Catania P N (1994). Home Health Care: The New Practice Site. *US Pharmacist* Supplement May, 3–10.

Chamberlain T M, Lehman M E, Groh M J, *et al.* (1998). Cost analysis of a home intravenous antibiotic program. *AJHP* 45: 2341–45.

Charles B (1990). Home Health Care in France. *Pharmaceutisch Weekblad – Scientific Edition* 12 (1): 23–25.

Collins J A, Skidmore M A, Melvin D B, *et al.* (1990). Home intravenous dobutamine therapy in patients awaiting heart transplantation. *J Heart Transplant* 9: 205–8.

Cote D, Oruck J, Thickson N (1989). A review of the Manitoba home IV antibiotic program. *Canadian J Hosp Pharm* 42: 137–41.

Curtis D (1997). Pontefract Hospitals NHS Trust: Interim evaluation of the hospital-at-home scheme pilot study. *JTQM* 8 (5): 205–10.

DeMoss C J (1980). Giving intravenous therapy at home. *Am J Nurs* 80: 2188–89.

Dies F, Krell M J, Whitlow P (1986). Intermittent dobutamine in ambulatory outpatients with chronic cardiac failure. *Circulation* 74(Suppl II): 38.

DoH (1998). *A first class service: quality in the new NHS.* London: The Stationery Office.

Dover S (1988). Advances in the use of opioids for domiciliary terminal care. *Practitioner* 232: 884–86.

Elia M (1995). An international perspective on artificial nutritional support in the community. *Lancet* 345(8961): 1345–49.

Gilbert J G T, Litlewood J M (1988). Home intravenous antibiotic treatment in cystic fibrosis. *Arch Dis Child* 63: 512–17.

Glick H A, Eisenberg J M, Koffer H, *et al.* (1991). Savings from faster return to nursing homes for patients hospitalised for infection. *Journal of Research in PharmacoEconomics* 3: 41–71.

Graham D R (1993). Nosohusial infections: a complication of home intravenous therapy. *Infect Dis Clin Pract* 2: 158–61.

Graham D R, Keldermans M M, Klemm L W, *et al.* (1991). Infectious complications among patients receiving home intravenous therapy with peripheral, central or peripherally placed central venous catheters. *AJM* 91(Suppl 3B): 95S–100S.

Grizzard M B, Harris G, Karns H (1991). Use of outpatient parenteral antibiotic therapy in a health maintenance organisation. *Reviews of Infectious Diseases* 13(Suppl 2): S174–S179.

Harries U, Hill S (1994). Measuring outcomes. *Health Service Journal* Sept 22: 25.

Hatwig C A (1996). Developing pharmacy's role in ambulatory care: Parkland Health and Hospital System. *Am J Health Syst Pharm* 53(Suppl 1): S27–S32.

Heizer W D, Orringer E P (1977). Parenteral nutrition at home for 4 years via arteriovenous fistulae. Supplemental intravenous feedings for a patient with severe short bowel syndrome. *Gastroenterology* 72: 527–32.

Jayabose S, Escobedo R N, Tugal O, *et al.* (1992). Home chemotherapy for children with cancer. *Cancer* 69(2): 574–79.

Jeejeebhoy K N (1973). Total parenteral nutrition at home for 23 months without complication and with good rehabilitation. *Gastroenterology* 65: 811–20.

Jennings P (1994). Learning through experience: an evaluation of 'Hospital at Home'. *J Adv Nurs* 19: 905–11.

Kayley J, Breendt A R, Snelling M J M, *et al.* (1996). Safe intravenous antibiotic therapy at home: experience of a UK based programme. *JAC*: 37 1023–29.

Kawaguchi Y, Tamura H, Hattori M, *et al.* (1994). Problems and solutions of home care for a terminal cancer patient. *Japanese Journal of Cancer and Chemotherapy* 21: 535–55.

Kind A C, Williams D N, Gibson J (1985). Outpatient intravenous antibiotic therapy – ten years experience. *Postgrad Med* 77(2): 105–11.

Knowelden J, Westlake L, Wright K G, *et al.* (1991). Peterborough hospital at home: an evaluation. *J Public Health Med* 13(30): 182–88.

Kunkel M J (1993). Outpatient parenteral antibiotic therapy. Management of serious infections. Part 1: medical, socioeconomic and legal issues. *Hosp Pract* 28(Suppl 1): 33–8.

Malloy J A (1990). Home Care Accreditation through Joint Commission on Accreditation of Healthcare Organisations. *Journal of Intravenous Nursing* 13(3): 185–87.

Malone M (1994). Quality of life of patients receiving home parenteral or enteral nutrition support. *PharmacoEconomics* 5(2): 101–8.

Marius-Nunez A L, Heaney L, Fernandez R N, *et al.* (1996). Intermittent inotropic therapy in an outpatient setting: a cost-effective therapeutic modality in patients with refractory heart failure. *Am Heart J* 132: 805–8.

McCorkle R, Jepson C, Malone D (1994). The impact of hospital home care on patients with cancer. *Res Nurs Health* 17: 243–51.

Monalto M, Grayson M L (1998). Acceptability of early discharge, hospital at home schemes (letter). *BMJ* 317: 1652.

Milkovich G (1995). Benefits of outpatient parenteral antibiotic therapy: to the individual, the institution, third party payers and society. *Int J Antimicrob Agents* 5: 27–31.

Miller L W, Merkle E J, Jennison S H (1994). Outpatient use of dobutamine to support patients awaiting heart transplantation. *J Heart Lung Transplant* 13: S126–S129.

Morales J O, Snead H (1994). Efficacy and safety of intravenous cefotaxime for treating pneumonia in outpatients. *AJM* 97: 28–33.

NAIT (1993). NAIT Report. *Am J Hosp Pharm* 50(May): 846–9.

New P B, Swanson G F, Bulich R G, *et al.* (1991). Ambulatory antibiotic infusion devices: Extending the spectrum of outpatient therapies. *AJM* 91: 455–61.

NHSiS Management Executive (1998). *Renewing the National Health Service in Scotland*. Guidance on Clinical Governance.

Nolet B (1989). Patient care issues in outpatient intravenous antibiotic therapy. *Infect Dis in Clin Pract* 3(3): 225–26.

Parker S E, Nathwani D, O'Reily D, *et al.* (1998). Evaluation of the impact of non-inpatient IV antibiotic treatment for acute infections on the hospital, primary care services and the patient. *JAC* 42: 373–80.

Phillips P (1992). Home dobutamine. *Canadian Nurse* 11: 13–15.

Poretz D M (1993). Infusion center, office and home. *Hosp Pract* 28(Suppl 2): 40–3.

Raehl C L, Bond C A, Pitterle M E (1993). Ambulatory pharmacy services affiliated with acute care hospitals. *Pharmacotherapy* 13(6): 618–25.

Rehm S J, Weinstein A J (1983). Home intravenous antibiotic therapy, a team approach. *Ann Intern Med* 99(3): 388–92.

Rich D (1994). Physicians, Pharmacists, and Home Infusion Antibiotic Therapy. *AJM* 97(Suppl 2A): 3–8.

Richards D M, Deeks J J, Sheldon T A, *et al.* (1997). Home parenteral nutrition: a systematic review. *Health Technol Assess* 1(1): i–iii, 1–59.

Rolston K V I (1995). Outpatient management of febrile, neutropenic patients. *Infect Med* 11: 12–15.

Rubinstein E (1993). Cost implications of home care on serious infections. *Hosp Form* 28(Suppl 1): 46–50.

Rucker R W, Harrison G M (1974). Outpatient intravenous medications in the management of cystic fibrosis. *Pediatrics* 54(3): 358–60.

Scully B E (1992). Home intravenous antibiotic therapy. *New Jersey Medicine*. 89(1): 48–51.

Secretary of State for Health (1997). *The new NHS: modern, dependable*. Cm 3807. London: The Stationery Office.

Secretary of State for Scotland (1997). *Designed to care. Renewing the NHS in Scotland*. Cm 3811. Edinburgh: The Stationery Office.

Sewell G, Bradford E, Rowland C G (1987). HOPE for cancer. *J Dist Nurs* April: 4–6.

Shane R (1996). Developing pharmacy's role in ambulatory care: Cedars-Sinai Medical Center. *Am J Health Syst Pharm* 53(Suppl 1): S32–S36.

Sharp J W (1986). Social work in a home intravenous antibiotic therapy program. *Soc Work Health Care* 12: 93–101.

Shaughnessy P J, Crisler K S, Kramer A M (1989). *Quality of care indicators in home care: preliminary indicators and directions for future research*. University of Colorado Health Sciences Centre, Denver.

Shils M E (1975). A program for total parenteral nutrition at home. *Am J Clin Nutr* 28: 1429–35.

Simmons B, Trusler M, Roccaforte J, *et al.* (1990). Infection control for home health. *Inf Control Hosp Epidemiol* 11: 362–70.

Sindone A P, Keogh A .M, Macdonald P S, *et al.* (1998). Continuous home ambulatory intravenous inotropic drug therapy in severe heart failure: safety and cost efficacy. *Am Heart J* 134(5): 889–900.

Stern S H, Singer L B, Weissman S E (1995). Analysis of hospital cost in total knee arthroplasty. Does length of stay matter? *Clin Orthop* 321: 36–44.

Stiver H G, Telford G O, Mossey J M, *et al.* (1978). Intravenous antibiotic therapy at home. *Ann Intern Med* 89(1): 690–93.

Stiver H G, Trosky S K, Cote D D, *et al.* (1982). Self-administration of intravenous antibiotics: an efficient, cost-effective home care program. *CMAJ* 127: 207–11.

Thickson N D (1993). Economics of home intravenous services. *PharmacoEconomics* 3: 220–27.

Tice A D (1991). Once daily ceftriaxone outpatient therapy in adults with infections. *Chemotherapy* 37(Suppl 3): 7–10.

Tice A D (1993). Growing pains in outpatient intravenous antibiotic therapy. *Infect Dis Clin Pract* 1: 74–6.

Tice A D (1996). Alternate site infusion. *JIN* 19(4): 188–93.

Watters C (1997). The benefits of providing chemotherapy at home. *Professional Nurse* 12(5): 367–70.

Wiernikowski J T, Rothney M, Dawson S, *et al.* (1991). Evaluation of a home intravenous antibiotic program in pediatric oncology. *American Journal of Pediatric Hematology and Oncology* 13: 144–47.

Williams D N, Bosch D, Boots J, *et al.* (1993). Safety, efficacy and cost savings in an outpatient intravenous antibiotic program. *Clin Ther* 15: 169–79.

Williams S E (1998). Personal communication. Department of General Practice and Primary Care, University of Aberdeen.

Wiselka M J, Nicholson K G (1997). Outpatient parenteral antimicrobial therapy: experience in a large teaching hospital. *J Infect* 35: 73–6.

8

Health promotion (I): smoking cessation

Hazel Sinclair

Introduction

Community pharmacists and health promotion

The community pharmacist's role has come full circle. Prior to the implementation in 1948 of the National Health Service Act 1946, the pharmacist was frequently the main source of medical advice for the less affluent (Sharpe, 1985). As had been the vision of Aneurin Bevan, the National Health Service aimed to bring a comprehensive medical service to all, irrespective of ability to pay, and the advisory role of the pharmacist subsequently declined. Unfortunately, the success of the NHS in keeping people alive into old age and new treatments resulting from advances in medical science, have caused costs to escalate. As a consequence, the Government has recognised the need to reduce the demand on the NHS and to give people greater responsibility for their own healthcare, and has adopted a new attitude to health promotion and self-medication (Nathan, 1995).

The fundamental aim of health promotion is to enable people to have more control over aspects of their lives which affect their health (WHO, 1984). The World Health Organization's succinct definition of health promotion encompasses two main features: improving health and being more in control of it: 'health promotion is the process of enabling people to increase control over, and to improve, their health' (WHO, 1984). While Downie *et al.*, define health promotion as an umbrella term: 'health promotion comprises efforts to enhance positive health and prevent ill-health, through the overlapping spheres of health education, prevention, and health protection' (Downie *et al.*, 1990), they also highlight empowerment, 'helping people to greater control over their lives and health'. The latter is a major principle of health promotion, emphasising the importance of two-way conversation where the 'providers' and 'recipients' each learn from each other, in contrast to the 'top down' or 'medically dominated' model (Downie *et al.*, 1990).

Community pharmacy services have the advantage over general practitioner (GP) services in being perceived by some customers as being more approachable and accessible (Jepson *et al.*, 1991; Williamson *et al.*, 1992; Vallis, 1994). A study of consultations demonstrated the pharmacist-client relationship as relatively equal, with no systematic pattern of domination by either the pharmacist or the customer (Smith, 1992). This relationship could facilitate health promotion, since the customer may feel more relaxed and able to raise concerns, ask for clarification of advice or challenge the recommendations of the pharmacist.

Smoking cessation

Cigarette smoking is the commonest cause of preventable morbidity and premature mortality in the UK, Europe and the developed world (Amos and Hillhouse, 1992) and has been described as causing a 'world-wide epidemic of death from tobacco' (Doll *et al.*, 1994). Smoking-related diseases account for 15–20% of all deaths in Britain and 431 000 deaths in the EC (WHO, 1991).

The extent of the damage to health caused by tobacco has been recognised by the Government and specific targets were set for reducing smoking by the year 2000 (Secretary of State for Health, 1992; Scottish Office, 1992). The Government stressed the central role of the primary healthcare team (PHCT) in helping to meet these targets, emphasising the importance of health education and co-ordinated action by a wide range of partners (HEBS, 1995). A role in smoking cessation for UK community pharmacy personnel is particularly appropriate because of the reclassification of nicotine replacement therapies (NRTs) from prescription-only medicines (POMs) to pharmacy (P) medicines, which means these treatments can be advertised to the general public and sold under the supervision of a pharmacist. Since 60% of the population visit a community pharmacy at least once a month (Institute of Pharmacy Management, 1991) pharmacy personnel (including both pharmacists and their assistants) are well placed to provide readily accessible support and encouragement to potential non-smokers and so facilitate informed decision making. However, despite health promotion being encouraged in community pharmacies through a contractual obligation for UK community pharmacists to display health promotion leaflets, over a quarter of users of NRT do not recall receiving any pharmacy counselling (Sinclair, 1995).

Following the change in status of NRTs, a vast array of support material (Anonymous, 1993; Anonymous, 1994) has been sent to pharmacies. The dissemination of guidelines in printed form alone has been shown to be ineffective in the medical setting (Russell and Grimshaw, 1992) and whilst there is no evidence to support an analogous behaviour in pharmacy, it seems more than likely that similar caveats would hold. The task of helping smokers to change their behaviour requires a particular set of skills and attitudes and most healthcare personnel are given little or no appropriate training (Rollnick, 1993). Moreover, in some pharmacies, advice on over-the-counter medicines is frequently provided by a pharmacy assistant (Hassell, 1996), who refers the customers to the pharmacist only when they believe they have insufficient knowledge or if the customer asks to speak to the pharmacist. It is therefore important that all members of the pharmacy team have the appropriate training to equip them with both the knowledge of medicines available and communication skills appropriate to the application of that knowledge to individual patient interactions (Evans and Moclair, 1994; Flint, 1995).

'Stage of change' model of behaviour change

A central principle of the self-empowerment approach to health promotion (WHO, 1984; Downie *et al.*, 1990) is understanding why people behave in certain ways and enabling them to change if they choose. Social psychology is a useful means of helping healthcare professionals understand how people conceptualise health and make decisions about their health and is therefore a useful tool in planning health promotion interventions (Naidoo and Wills, 1994; National Heart Forum, 1995). Several models of behaviour change have been developed in an attempt to explain the influence of different variables on a person's health-related behaviour (Naidoo and Wills, 1994; National Heart Forum, 1995). The 'stage of change' model of behaviour change (Prochaska and DiClemente, 1983; Prochaska and Goldstein, 1991) has been used widely and successfully in American work with drug, alcohol and gambling addiction. However, further work was needed to confirm the superiority of the model (Ashworth, 1997) and to demonstrate its utility on a wider geographic scale and in different professional contexts.

Recent work has underlined the importance of willingness to change, by showing that motivation rather than technique is a major determinant of successful smoking cessation (Lennox and Taylor,

1994; Sinclair *et al.*, 1995). The model emphasises the importance of the individual's degree of readiness to change, a sentiment echoed by Naidoo and Wills (1994): 'there is a clear message for those health educators who work with individual clients and who are sometimes accused of 'telling people what to do'; people will only change if they want to.'

The 'stage of change' model identifies six stages: precontemplation, contemplation, preparation, action, maintenance and relapse. Progress through the stages is cyclical rather than linear (Figure 8.1), and at each stage people need different types of support and advice. People seeking help with smoking cessation from community pharmacy personnel are already beyond the precontemplation stage and will have reached the contemplation or preparation stage. Many may be intending to purchase an anti-smoking aid. For smokers who decide to stop smoking, NRT increases the chance of success (Sutherland *et al.*, 1992; Mant and Fowler, 1993; Tang *et al.*, 1994). An understanding of the theory and practice of the model could promote more effective counselling by helping pharmacy personnel to tailor their advice to the stage the customer is at, which may in turn be expected to optimise the potential of any therapy. In particular, the use of the 'stage of change' model by pharmacy personnel could:

- Help move smokers from the contemplation and preparation stage to the action and maintenance stages where the use of NRT is appropriate.
- Improve the effectiveness of the treatment by reducing inappropriate use of NRT by targeting it to smokers at the correct stages of the model.
- Increase the chance of smoking cessation success by providing important additional support matched to the need of the individual.
- Encourage customers who lapse to try again when they feel ready by remaining supportive and positive.
- Be more effective in terms of time by reducing inappropriate intervention.

The research question and methods

Smoking cessation training for community pharmacy

Despite the supervision of NRT sales having moved rapidly from the general practitioner to the pharmacist (Sinclair *et al.*, 1995) and, despite the participation of pharmacists in health education campaigns, there have been no controlled trials of the effectiveness of intervention by

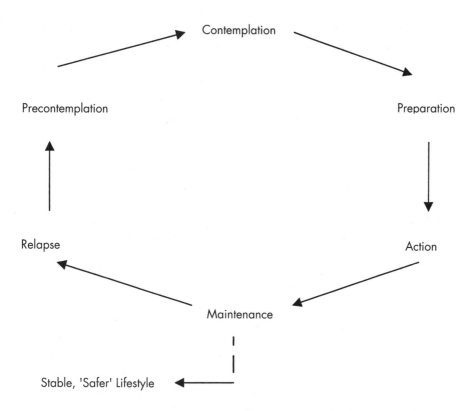

Figure 8.1 'Stage of Change' model of behaviour change (Prochaska and DiClemente, 1983)

pharmacy personnel on the sale of non-prescription medicines (Berbatis, 1991). Moreover, most NRT users would like to have more pharmacy support, in particular, regular individual counselling (Sinclair *et al.*, 1995). In the autumn of 1994, it was therefore decided that there was a need to develop an effective training programme for pharmacy personnel in order to offer a free, ongoing counselling service to customers, to monitor the outcome of this training using a pragmatic study on a sample representative of the population of smokers who are seeking advice in the pharmacy and/or are purchasing anti-smoking products, and to assess the cost-effectiveness of such a pharmacy intervention.

A two-hour training package, based on the 'stage of change' model of smoking cessation (Prochaska and DiClemente, 1983; Prochaska and

Goldstein, 1991), was commissioned from Grampian Health Promotions by the Department of General Practice and Primary Care at the University of Aberdeen and the School of Pharmacy at the Robert Gordon University. Unlike similar training for hospital doctors (Goldberg *et al.*, 1994), for general practitioners and practice nurses (Stott *et al.*, 1995), and for general practitioners, practice nurses and health visitors (Lennox *et al.*, 1996), the training did not include motivational interviewing techniques to encourage smokers to move from precontemplation to contemplation. However, it did include specific content and recommendations pertaining to the maintenance and relapse stages of the model. The training focused on the model using case studies of pharmacy customers, and on communication skills for negotiating change and providing ongoing support and encouragement tailored to the customer's current stage; it did not focus on NRT products. The training was piloted in mid-December 1994 on a cross-section of pharmacy personnel from outside the study sample.

The evaluation of the training intervention

Naidoo and Wills emphasise the importance of evaluation: 'Evaluation is necessary to the ongoing survival and viability of health promotion. To compete successfully for resources in today's economic climate, health promoters must be able to demonstrate hard results. It is not good enough to have good intentions' (Naidoo and Wills, 1994).

The research question was therefore whether providing training to community pharmacy personnel would improve the smoking cessation outcome of customers they advised.

The remainder of this section describes the evaluation of the training initiative for pharmacists and pharmacy assistants, based on the 'stage of change' model, which aimed to increase smoking cessation success rates in the community pharmacy setting in Grampian, Scotland, by improving the counselling offered by pharmacy personnel. However, the scope of the evaluation was not limited to the binary measure of smoking cessation outcome, but adopted a multiple-method approach using both quantitative and qualitative techniques to look in depth at the impact of the training and the process of the pharmacy support. A comprehensive economic evaluation was also built into the study. Pluralistic evaluation was adopted and so the views of pharmacists, pharmacy assistants and customers were reported.

Selection of the method

The advantages and drawbacks of three broad types of study were considered before deciding on a randomised controlled trial (RCT) as the most appropriate technique to evaluate the training as shown in Figure 8.2.

Randomised controlled trials are the best way to compare the effectiveness of different interventions (Altman, 1996). The random allocation of the participant pharmacies to either the test or control group meant that the groups should be exactly similar in all respects prior to the intervention, and so gave the potential to provide the most powerful evidence of cause and effect by evaluating the intervention against a control which continued to provide standard professional pharmaceutical support. The RCT design allowed the conditions to be under the direct control of the researcher and was the easiest method to remove bias and minimise the susceptibility to confounding. Moreover, randomisation meant that a post-test only design was all that was required for a true experiment, thus avoiding the problematic effects of a pre-test to take measures before the experiment (Campbell and Stanley, 1963).

Process and outcome measures

The study aimed to address the three main reasons identified by Downie, Fyfe and Tannahill for evaluating health programmes. To avoid discouraging results, evaluation should be appropriate to the stage of development of the health promotion initiative (Downie *et al.*, 1990). Although smoking cessation outcome was a major long-term evaluation measure, with the intervention being in its early stages of development,

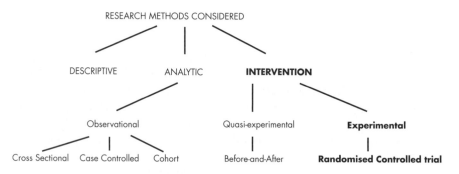

Figure 8.2 Selection of method

priority was also given to the evaluation of the process of the health promotion in order to ascertain at what point failure had occurred should the RCT show no difference between the smoking cessation rates of the groups.

The following outcome measures were used to evaluate the operation of the programme (process), its short-term effects (impact) and its long-term effects (outcome); see p. 79 for Notes:

- customers' self-reported point prevalence at one month[1] (outcome);
- customers' self-reported continuous abstinence of four months and nine months[1] (outcome);
- pharmacy personnel's perceptions of the value and utility of the training package (impact, process and outcome);
- customers' perceptions of the support provided by pharmacy personnel (process);
- pharmacist and pharmacy assistants KS[2], ES[3] and OS[4], at two, 12, 24 and 36 months after the training (outcome);
- average pharmacy KS, ES, and OS (PKS[5], PES[6] and POS[7]), at two, 12, 24 and 36 months after the training (outcome).

Consideration was given to the validation of self-reported measurements of smoking status using biochemical markers, such as exhaled carbon monoxide or blood and salivary measurements of nicotine metabolites. However, it was decided to rely on self-reported smoking status, since a comprehensive review of the subject by Velicer *et al.* (1992) concluded that biochemical validation was not indicated for this type of brief intervention:

> 'the scientific benefits of trying to validate self-reported measures of smoking status are often not worth the tremendous practical costs. In most studies, there would not be large enough samples to demonstrate significant differences in false reporting rates, even if one group has twice as much false reporting as the other group.' (Velicer *et al.* 1992).

Ethics

The Joint Ethical Committee of Grampian Health Board and the University of Aberdeen requires researchers to provide a patient information sheet outlining the study and informing patients that they are free both to refuse to participate and to withdraw at any stage. The study protocol was approved by the Joint Ethical Committee, and the patient information sheets complied with the Code of Ethics of the Royal Pharmaceutical Society of Great Britain (RPSGB).

The study

Subjects

Pharmacy personnel

In September 1994, all of the 76 non-city (Aberdeen) community pharmacies registered in Grampian Region were sent an outline of the study and were invited to participate in a randomised controlled trial to test the effectiveness of the training. The city pharmacies were excluded to prevent contaminating a similar training initiative for general practitioners and practice staff in Aberdeen city (Lennox *et al.*, 1996). Non-respondent pharmacies were sent a reminder after three weeks and were followed up by telephone after a further three weeks. Pharmacy recruits were stratified by type (national multiple or proprietor owned) and ranked according to the pharmacist's level of motivation (as defined by the date their 'willingness to participate' proforma was received). They were then randomised to either the intervention or control group by sequential allocation. All the intervention pharmacists and pharmacy assistants who were routinely involved in giving anti-smoking advice and/or the sale of NRT products were invited to attend the training in January 1995. The control pharmacies were contacted by telephone and asked to provide the names of all their personnel who dealt routinely with anti-smoking enquiries or sales.

Customers

During the 12-month recruitment period, all smokers who sought advice on stopping smoking and/or, in preparation for a new attempt to stop smoking, presented a private prescription or bought an anti-smoking product over the counter, were eligible for inclusion. Pharmacy personnel offered these customers a patient information sheet inviting them to join the study. Customers who were willing to participate then registered with that pharmacy, so joining either the intervention or control group as determined by the group to which that pharmacy had been allocated. To monitor non-recruitment, pharmacies in both groups maintained a tally record of customers who declined to join the study, and their reasons.

Sample size

The determinant of sample size was continuous abstinence at the nine-month follow-up; this was also the measure likely to show the smallest difference between the intervention and control groups. The most comparable data on outcome in a pharmacy setting reported 15% not smoking at one month and 9% at seven months (assuming non-responders had lapsed) (Sinclair *et al.*, 1995). This was used to estimate a control group continuous abstinence rate of 7% at nine months. A worthwhile effect of the training intervention was taken as a 5% increase in this figure to 12% for the subjects exposed to the effect of the intervention. Assuming subjects lost to follow-up had lapsed, the number of subjects required to detect a 5% improvement with a power of 80% and a probability of 95% was determined using the formula for calculating sample size for unpaired proportions (Russell, 1984). At least 538 subjects were required in each group to give an 80% chance of detecting a 5% difference in smoking cessation success rate (from 7% to 12%) which is statistically significant at the 5% level (two-tailed test).

Study design

A multi-stage design was used to evaluate the training, with seven pharmacy stages and five customer stages as shown in Table 8.1.

Pharmacy stages

In the initial stage, the researcher participated as an observer (Baker, 1994), taking field notes during the workshop of pharmacy participant interactions and of issues raised. The second stage assessed the immediate impact of the training on the workshop participants using the Workshop Impact Questionnaire. In the third stage, both groups completed a Knowledge and Attitude Questionnaire two months after the training. The fourth, sixth and seventh stages used the same Knowledge and Attitude Questionnaire to assess the level of decay in knowledge (Downie *et al.*, 1990) and to monitor changes in attitude after 12, 24 and 36 months. Sixteen months after the training, the intervention personnel available for follow up were each contacted by post and invited to participate in a telephone interview (fifth stage). A quota sample of 20 personnel was selected from those willing to be interviewed; the sample aimed to reflect the range of characteristics: age, gender, staff grade (pharmacist/assistant), smoking status, and multiple/non-multiple location. The interviews aimed to gather in-depth information on the pharmacy personnel's perceptions of the value and utility of the training and to identify constraints to its implementation.

Table 8.1 Pharmacy stages

Stage	Data collection method	Subjects	Timing
1	Observation by researcher	All workshop participants	during workshop 0 months
2	Workshop Impact Questionnaire (self-completion)	All workshop participants	end of workshop 0 months
3	Knowledge and Attitude Questionnaire (postal, self-completion)	All available workshop participants, and control personnel who routinely gave advice on stopping smoking and/or handled NRT sales	at 2 months
4	Knowledge and Attitude Questionnaire (postal, self-completion)	All available workshop participants and control personnel (as Stage 3 above)	at 12 months
5	Semi-Structured Interview with researcher (telephone)	Quota-sample (n = 20) of intervention personnel selected from those willing to participate in an interview	at 18 months
6	Knowledge and Attitude Questionnaire (postal, self-completion)	All available workshop participants and control personnel (as Stage 3 above)	at 24 months
7	Knowledge and Attitude Questionnaire (postal, self-completion)	All available workshop participants and control personnel (as Stage 3 above)	at 36 months

Customer stages

Customers completed a Registration Postcard Questionnaire in the pharmacy and were followed up by postal questionnaires at one, four and nine months. As part of the One Month Questionnaire, all the subjects were requested to give a daytime and/or evening contact telephone number if they would be willing to participate in a follow-up telephone interview six months after registration (fourth stage). A sub-sample of 25 intervention interviewees and 25 controls was selected using stratified sampling in conjunction with systematic sampling (Baker, 1994). Customers who provided a contact number were stratified by group and ranked by date of recruitment, then every fourth subject was selected for interview. The interviews aimed to validate four-month questionnaire data and collect in depth information on the customers' perceptions of the support provided in the pharmacy. These stages are summarised in Table 8.2.

Data collection

Methods

A combination of methods was used. This pluralistic method of enquiry used observation, self-administered questionnaires and semi-structured telephone interviews to gain from the strengths of each method while compensating for the limitations of each approach. This is shown in Table 8.3.

Data collection instruments

Pharmacy The Workshop Impact Questionnaire was developed to monitor the participants' immediate impressions of the workshop. A four-point Likert rating scale (from 'very poor' to 'very good') was used to assess the workshop as a learning experience and as a use of the participant's time. Another four-point rating scale (from 'No' to 'Yes') monitored whether the respondents felt they had been encouraged to participate during the workshop and whether they felt they would be able to use what they had learned. The questionnaire was pre-tested during the pilot workshops.

A literature review failed to identify any appropriate validated rating scale to evaluate the effect of the training on participants. It was therefore decided to develop a self-rated attitudinal scale to evaluate the participants' knowledge and understanding of, and belief in, the 'stage of change' model (knowledge (K)), their confidence in their own ability to counsel smokers (self-efficacy (E)) and their perceived outcome of pharmacy counselling on smoking cessation (outcome (O)). Full details of the questionnaire, the scoring system for the rating scales, and the piloting and validation of the instrument are reported elsewhere (Sinclair *et al.*, 1998a).

An interview topic guide was developed in order to gather in depth information on the perceived value of the training, to identify constraints to its implementation, and to differentiate between the training needs of the pharmacist as opposed to their assistants. The topic guide was pre-tested on two pharmacists and two assistants from the intervention group.

Customer The Registration Postcard recorded the subject's name and contact address, whether an anti-smoking product was purchased and,

Table 8.2 Customer stages

Stage	Data collection method	Subjects	Timing
1	Registration Questionnaire (self-completion)	All customers who sought anti-smoking advice and/or bought an anti-smoking product at the start of a new attempt to stop smoking	On recruitment
2	One-Month Questionnaire (postal, self-completion)	All available for follow-up	1 month after recruitment
3	Four-Month Questionnaire (postal, self-completion)	All available for follow-up	4 months after recruitment
4	Semi-Structured Interview with researcher (telephone)	Sub-sample (25 intervention, 25 controls) selected from those willing to participate	6 months after recruitment
5	Nine-Month Questionnaire (postal, self-completion)	All who had not previously indicated they had lapsed	9 months after recruitment

Table 8.3 Quantitative and qualitative methods: strengths and limitations[a]

Method	Strengths	Limitations
Survey questionnaires	Data on a large number of subjects can be collected efficiently Precise comparisons can be made between the answers given by different respondents	Limited depth Questions are in a highly standardised format Self-completion – no opportunity for verbal clarification
Telephone interviews	In-depth data Rich source of data	Lower numbers due to time and financial costs More difficult to compare with other studies and to generalise Influence of interviewer
Observation	In-depth data Rich source of data Participants interact and fresh slants are uncovered	Limited numbers May be dominated by hierarchy within participants Bias caused by researcher presence Bias caused by researcher judgement

[a] Data sources: Baker, 1994; Farmer and Miller, 1994.

if so, the name of the product. The One-Month Questionnaire monitored self-reported smoking status (point prevalence), it recorded demographic characteristics (gender, age, postcode (a proxy for economic
deprivation (Carstairs and Morris, 1991)), and previous nicotine dependence (Heatherton *et al.*, 1991)). Information was also sought on the
subject's experience in the pharmacy when they first bought the product
as part of their current attempt to stop smoking (for example, whether
they were questioned regarding current health status or advised on
product strength and use). The Four-Month Questionnaire monitored
self-reported continuous abstinence from zero to four months and the
customers' perceptions of the support they received from pharmacy
personnel. The Nine-Month Questionnaire monitored self-reported continuous abstinence from zero to nine months.

A telephone interview topic guide was developed to validate the
Four-Month Questionnaire data and obtain in-depth information on the
customers' experiences of the pharmacy counselling and support
received. Data were also gathered on the duration of the initial and subsequent consultations. Finally, willingness to pay (WTP) (Donaldson *et
al.*, 1995) was used to monitor the customers' perceptions of the monetary value of the pharmacy counselling they had received. Further information on willingness to pay is included in Chapter 4. The initial pilot
highlighted problems in using an open-ended approach to WTP. A
further pilot using a novel flexible payment scale confirmed the utility of
this alternative approach. This monitored the customers' perceptions of
the value of the pharmacy service they had actually received as a proportion of the weekly sum they paid for NRT (thus the upper value of
the scale was determined by the customer).

Data handling and analysis

Permission was sought from the interviewees to tape the telephone
interviews. The tapes were transcribed in full and the text read several
times to facilitate the identification of themes, quotes were then highlighted and grouped by theme. A computer software package, SPSS©
for Windows 6.1.3 (1995) was used to store and analyse questionnaire
data, to calculate descriptive statistics, and to demonstrate differences
between the intervention and control groups using parametric tests
(t-tests for quantitative variables) and non-parametric tests (Mann-
Whitney tests for quantitative and chi-square test of association for
qualitative variables). Multiple logistic regression was carried out
(Dixon, 1993) for the binary outcomes of point prevalence at one

month, and continuous abstinence at four and nine months, and to assess the effect of potential confounders (age, sex, economic deprivation (Carstairs and Morris, 1991), and nicotine dependency (Heatherton *et al.*, 1991)). The effect of cluster randomisation was assessed by first calculating the degree of intra-cluster correlation (i.e. within pharmacy correlation) for each of the binary outcomes of abstinence. Secondly, regression techniques, adding the pharmacy as a

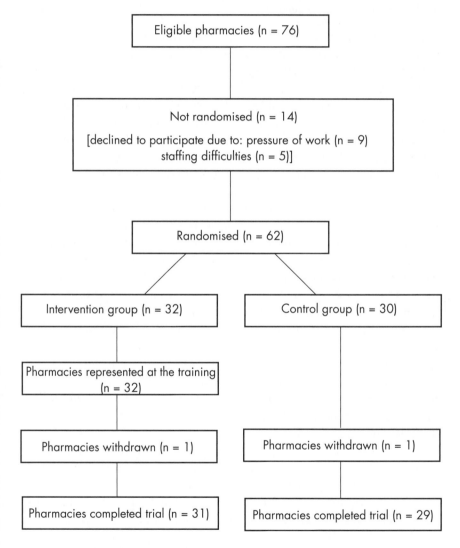

Figure 8.3 Flow diagram: community pharmacies (Sinclair *et al.* (1998b). *Tob Control* 7: 253–61, with permission from BMJ Publishing Group)

random factor nested within the treatment groups (intervention and control) to the other fixed effect factors, were considered leading to a generalised linear mixed model (GLMM) approach (Collett, 1991; Genstat, 1993).

Results

Participant flow and follow-up

The CONSORT statement (Altman, 1996) recommends the inclusion of a flow chart to describe the progress of subjects through randomised controlled trials. As shown in Figure 8.3 (Sinclair et al., 1998b), 62 pharmacies were recruited to the study, a recruitment rate of 82% (62/76) (intervention (n = 31) control (n = 31)). During the training it was noted that one intervention pharmacist was also in charge of an outlet allocated to the control group. This pharmacy was transferred to the intervention group. During the 12-month customer recruitment period, one control pharmacy withdrew due to pressure of work and one intervention pharmacy withdrew because of major staff changes (no customers had been recruited by either of these pharmacies). Thus, 31 intervention and 29 control pharmacies participated in the study.

All of the intervention pharmacies were represented at the training, and a total of 94 personnel participated (54 assistants, 40 pharmacists). The control pharmacies identified 120 personnel (80 assistants, 40 pharmacists) who routinely dealt with anti-smoking enquiries or sales. Figure 8.4 shows the flow diagram for community pharmacy personnel detailing the attrition of the initial population of pharmacy personnel and the response rates during the three year follow-up period.

The study recruited 492 subjects (224 intervention, 268 controls) from a total of 775 eligible customers; an overall recruitment rate of 64%. Detailed information on recruitment, non-recruitment and follow up at the three time points is given in the flow diagram shown in Figure 8.5 (Sinclair et al., 1998b).

The main outcome measure was nine months' continuous abstinence, so the 106 intervention and 136 control subjects who were already identified as smoking were not followed up at nine months. Thus nine-month self-reported smoking data were available for a total of 73% (347) of the recruited subjects: 73% (159) intervention and 73% (188) controls.

Analysis

Smoking cessation outcomes   Assuming non-responders had lapsed, one-month point prevalence was claimed by 37% (81) intervention and

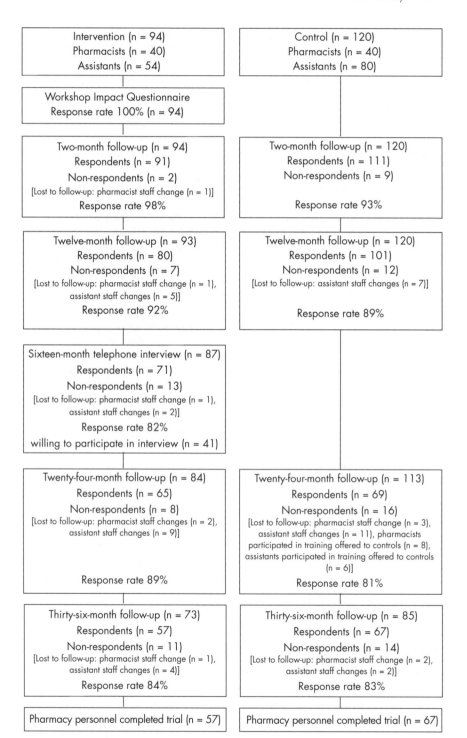

Figure 8.4 Flow diagram for community pharmacy personnel

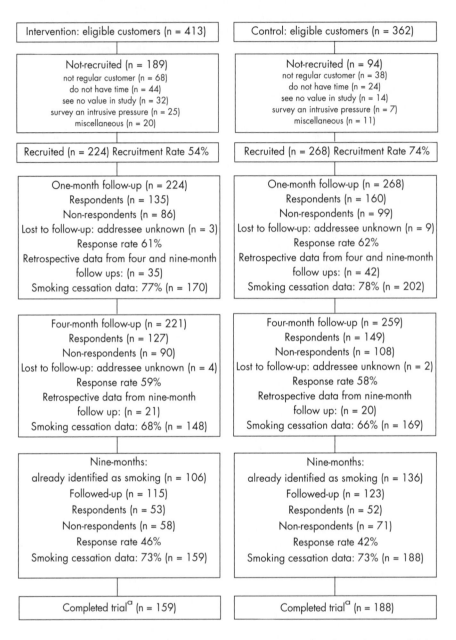

Figure 8.5 Flow diagram for customers ᵃi.e. nine-month smoking data available. (Reproduced with permission from Sinclair *et al.*, 1998b.)

29% (74) controls (p = 0.059); four months' continuous abstinence was claimed by 20% (44) intervention and 13% (32) controls (p = 0.021); and nine months' continuous abstinence by 12% (26) intervention and

7% (19) controls (p = 0.089). These differences were robust to confounders and to adjustment for clustering (Sinclair, 1997).

*Pharmacy personnel's perceptions of the value and utility of the train-
ing* The Workshop Impact Questionnaire demonstrated that 95% of
the participants rated the workshop as a 'good' or 'very good' learning
experience and a 'good' or 'very good' use of their time, and that 90%
thought they would be able to utilise what they had learned at the workshop in their work. By the two-month follow up, 82% of the workshop
participants had utilised the training, 90% by 12 months. The most
frequently cited reasons for not utilising the training was the lack of
relevant customers, and assistants who had referred the customers to
the pharmacist. The telephone interviews revealed that the majority of
pharmacists and assistants were extremely positive about the training;
in particular, it fulfilled a training need, was a more effective training
method, and provided information and a new understanding of the
psychological background of smokers. Almost all felt the training had
helped them to help their customers, by providing an orderly approach,
and a greater understanding and empathy towards smokers. It also
increased counsellor confidence and the incidence of counselling. Moreover, the majority felt the training had increased their job satisfaction
through their interaction with customers. Half had not encountered any
problems when asking local customers to register with the pharmacy;
however, difficulties were encountered by half the interviewees, in particular, customer reticence, and customer and pharmacy time constraints. Almost all were positive about counselling. However, in
practice, many factors interacted to influence counselling, for example,
the smoker's perceived need for support, commercial advertising, time,
and the commercial setting. Interviewees were less enthusiastic about
the records than the counselling; problems focused around customer
aversion towards the formality of the record, lack of customer commitment, and pharmacy factors (time, privacy, part-time staff). Further
detailed results are reported elsewhere (Sinclair, 1997; Sinclair *et al.*,
1998a).

*Customers' perceptions of the support provided by pharmacy person-
nel* The one-month questionnaire revealed that the intervention
respondents were significantly more likely to have discussed stopping
smoking with pharmacy personnel, 85% (113) compared with 62%
(99) of the controls (p = 0.000 01). They also rated their discussion
more highly; 34% (45) intervention compared with 16% (25) controls
rated it as 'very useful' (p = 0.048). At the time of their initial purchase,

intervention respondents were significantly more likely to have been asked about their health, 63% (83) compared with 45% (68) controls (p = 0.002 5), and advised on the strength of NRT, 89% (117) compared with 75% (112) controls (p = 0.003 7). The four-month questionnaire showed that 60% of the intervention respondents felt the pharmacy counselling had been helpful and that 40% found it helpful to know that the pharmacy was keeping a record of their progress. The majority of respondents had previously tried to stop smoking using an anti-smoking product; when asked to compare the current pharmacy support with previous attempt/s the intervention respondents were significantly more likely to rate their current support as 'better', while the controls rated it the 'same' (p = 0.000 64). The majority of telephone interviewees felt it was helpful to always use the same pharmacy because it encouraged the development of a long-term supportive relationship with pharmacy personnel. Others felt it made 'no difference' because pharmacies were equally good or, after learning about the product during the initial consultation, any pharmacy could be used for refill supplies. None of the interviewees mentioned dissatisfaction with regard to which member/s of the pharmacy team provided the counselling. Almost half were counselled by both the pharmacist and the assistants, the counter assistant was the only point of contact for over a quarter of interviewees, while a quarter were only counselled by the pharmacist. The majority appreciated on-going product advice and friendly interest and encouragement. Several highlighted personal motivation as the most important factor in stopping smoking; however, encouragement from pharmacy personnel was a useful adjunct. Several who had used NRT previously felt further advice had not made any difference; three control customers felt counselling was unwelcome and unhelpful. Half the intervention interviewees felt the record provided additional encouragement; however, one had mixed feelings ranging from encouraging to embarrassing. Many highlighted a lack of communication during previous attempts, with the prevailing attitude having been 'just another sale'. Customers particularly valued talking to the pharmacy personnel to gain information on the various products and the personal interest taken in their attempt. Further detailed results are reported elsewhere (Sinclair, 1997; Sinclair et al., 1998b).

Pharmacy personnel's knowledge and attitudes   The training had a significant effect on knowledge for at least three years, since at all four time points the intervention pharmacy teams had a greater knowledge and understanding of the model than the controls (2 months: p = 0.000 01;

12 months: p = 0.000 01; 24 months: p = 0.000 01; 36 months: p = 0.031). The first three follow-ups demonstrated that the intervention teams were also significantly more confident in their own ability to counsel customers (2 months: p = 0.046; 12 months: p = 0.026; 24 months: p = 0.021) and were more positive about the outcome of smoking cessation counselling provided in community pharmacies (2 months: p = 0.022; 12 months: p = 0.069; 24 months: p = 0.043) than their control counterparts. These attitudinal differences were no longer statistically significant at 36 months. The study also demonstrated that the training had a particularly positive effect on the knowledge and attitudes of the assistants. Further detailed results are reported elsewhere (Sinclair, 1997; Sinclair *et al.*, 1998a; Sinclair *et al.*, 1999a).

Economic evaluation

The greatest cost of the intervention, the retail price of the anti-smoking products, was borne by the customers. Correcting for the different group sizes, the intervention resulted in ten extra quitters at a marginal cost of £302 per quitter. Finally, the WTP data demonstrated that the intervention customers valued the advice they had received from pharmacy personnel more highly than the controls, 48% and 32% of their weekly cost of NRT respectively (p = 0.07). More detailed economic results are reported elsewhere (Sinclair *et al.*, 1999b).

Conclusions

Methodological strengths and weaknesses

A recent systematic review of randomised controlled trials on the effectiveness of training health professionals to provide smoking cessation interventions failed to identify any involving pharmacists (Silagy *et al.*, 1997). This is the first such study to report the effectiveness of smoking cessation training for pharmacy personnel.

Ideally, evaluation should be conducted by an objective outsider, since those directly involved in the development and delivery of the training would be likely to have a vested interest in the outcome of the evaluation (van Teijlingen *et al.*, 1995). Grampian Health Promotions developed and delivered the training, whilst the evaluation was primarily conducted by the Department of General Practice and Primary Care, University of Aberdeen, with additional support on pharmacy practice from the School of Pharmacy, Robert Gordon University, and economic expertise from the Health Economics Research Unit, University of Aberdeen. Thus, the main architects of the training were effectively removed from its evaluation.

Randomisation was by pharmacy rather than by customer, so minimising contamination between the groups; however, this cluster design meant that it could not be assumed that all individuals included in the analysis were independent, and so the degree of intracluster correlation was calculated; this was found to be negligible so the results could be treated as if randomised by customer.

The series of strategies used to maximise pharmacy recruitment, customer recruitment and both pharmacy and customer response rates proved to be effective, and so optimised the generalisability of the results. The study provided hard data on the effect of the intervention, the main outcome measure being the comparison of the smoking cessation rates of the intervention and control group customers at three time points. Cessation rates were reported on the basis of the standard assumption that non-responders had lapsed, so allowing comparisons to be made with other studies; this had the additional advantage that the power of the study was maintained with no missing values for the outcome measures. In order to monitor any relationship between intervention and control customers with respect to the potential confounders of age, sex, deprivation and nicotine dependency, multiple logistic regression analysis was carried out for the binary outcomes of point prevalence of abstinence at one month, and continuous abstinence at four and nine months.

The scope of the investigation was not limited to the binary measures of smoking cessation outcome. It adopted a multiple-method approach to look in depth at the impact of the training and the process of the pharmacy support. Pluralistic evaluation was adopted and so the views of pharmacists, pharmacy assistants and customers were reported.

The study suffered from several methodological weaknesses. Firstly, the decision to conduct the study in Grampian when a similar study was being conducted in Aberdeen city necessitated the exclusion of city pharmacies to prevent cross contamination and could have limited the generalisability of the results because of the under representation of urban outlets and large multiples in the pharmacy sample. Moreover, it was then likely that the sample of customers would also be unrepresentative of the general population of smokers who sought advice in pharmacies or bought anti-smoking products. However, despite these potential biasing factors, it appears that the study did in fact recruit a sample representative of the population of Scottish NRT users (Sinclair, 1997).

Secondly, in common with previously reported pharmacy practice research, this study failed to recruit all the eligible customers; in particular, intervention customers were reticent to join the study. However, analysis showed that the two arms of the study were well balanced at baseline and at each of the follow-ups in terms of the potential confounders of age, sex, affluence and nicotine dependency (Sinclair, 1997). Finally, it would have been preferable to have had a longer term outcome measure than nine months' continuous abstinence.

Implications for future practice

The investigation met its overall aim and each of the specific research objectives. Despite the bias of the pharmacy population towards more rural outlets, these results for Grampian have potential generalisability to the whole of Scotland since the population of customers was representative of the national population of NRT users (Sinclair, 1997).

The study validated the utility, in a Grampian community pharmacy setting, of training based on the 'stage of change' model of smoking behaviour change. It quantified the important contribution that appropriately trained community pharmacists and their assistants can make to achieving national smoking cessation targets. It demonstrated that an interactive training workshop is an effective means of teaching community pharmacists and pharmacy assistants the theory and practice of the model and that trained personnel were subsequently more effective than untrained controls in helping people, who had already reached the contemplation stage, to stop smoking and more of their customers claimed to have achieved nine months' abstinence.

The study identified a need for training on general issues relating to smoking, in particular the psychological background of smokers, instead of a product-based approach. The trained personnel thought the model was a good way of understanding stopping smoking. The majority reported they had utilised the training and felt it had made a difference to the way they counselled customers and had helped them to help their customers, which led to increased job satisfaction throughout the pharmacy team.

The study showed that the training had a significant effect on the participants' knowledge for at least three years and a significant effect on attitudes for two years. This could be an indication of the need for refresher training, but could also be attributed to the reduced power of the study due to attrition of the pharmacy sample. It confirmed the key role of counter assistants in providing advice on over-the-counter medicines and demonstrated the particularly positive effect of the training on the knowledge and attitudes of the assistants.

The Government, in its efforts to control the demand on the NHS, is encouraging health promotional activities (Secretary of State for Health, 1992; Scottish Office, 1992; Secretary of State for Health, 1998), is actively backing the increasing range of non-prescription medicines (Nathan, 1995; Bond and Bradley, 1996), and so is shifting the responsibility for the decision making process back to the individual. Thus, the patient assumes the responsibility of his/her own doctor. The study demonstrated that all levels of pharmacy personnel have the potential to be pharmacy facilitators, offering a value added service to help the patient-as-doctor make an informed choice about their use of pharmacy-only medicines. Intervention customers reported increased and more useful counselling. They were significantly more likely to feel that the pharmacy support had improved and they valued the support significantly higher in monetary terms than their control counterparts. Although both customers and pharmacy personnel were more positive about the counselling than the client records, ways of publicising new services to customers should be developed since a significant number of intervention customers felt the records had been an additional encouragement. Pharmacy personnel should offer support but also be sensitive to the wishes of the minority of customers who prefer to make an autonomous purchase without any input from the pharmacy.

The study confirmed that females are higher users of over-the-counter anti-smoking products than men and that the prognosis for females attempting to stop smoking, with the aid of NRT bought from community pharmacies, is encouraging (Sinclair, 1997). However, despite the inverse relationship between socio-economic group and smoking, the study confirmed the greater use of NRT by the more affluent and so it appears that the intervention was less effective in reaching poorer smokers (Sinclair, 1997).

The intervention personnel were less likely to classify customers who lapsed as failures (Sinclair *et al.*, 1998a; Sinclair *et al.*, 1999). It could therefore be expected that a more long-term effect of the training would be that these customers would encounter a more understanding and encouraging attitude if they returned to the pharmacy as part of a further attempt to stop smoking. This is a particularly important point given the customer sensitivity identified during the study.

The wider adoption of this training programme for pharmacists and pharmacy assistants would be expected to increase the potential of NRT and make a significant contribution to achieving national smoking cessation targets at a minimal cost to the NHS, since the major cost of the intervention, the retail price of the anti-smoking products, was borne by the customers.

The consultation on the future of the profession, led by the Royal Pharmaceutical Society of Great Britain (RPSGB, 1995; RPSGB, 1996), has highlighted the need for positive action to realise the potential of pharmacy and so increase its contribution to patient care. The findings from this study are encouraging, confirming that appropriately trained pharmacy personnel can offer better support to people who are attempting to change to, and maintain, a healthier lifestyle.

Notes

1. Adopting the normal convention (National Heart Forum, 1995), it was assumed that all non-responders had lapsed.
2. Knowledge Score: a measure of pharmacy personnel's knowledge and understanding of the 'stage of change' model.
3. Efficacy Score: a measure of pharmacy personnel's perceived self-efficacy to counsel smokers.
4. Outcome Score: a measure of pharmacy personnel's perceptions of the outcome of smoking cessation counselling in the pharmacy.
5. Pharmacy Knowledge Score: the average KS of all the personnel in a single pharmacy who counsel customers on stopping smoking and/or handle NRT sales.
6. Pharmacy Efficacy Score: the average ES of all the personnel in a single pharmacy who counsel customers on stopping smoking and/or handle NRT sales.
7. Pharmacy Outcome Score: the average OS of all the personnel in a single pharmacy who counsel customers on stopping smoking and/or handle NRT sales.

Acknowledgements

Crown copyright material is reproduced with the permission of the Controller of Her Majesty's Stationery Office, the BMJ Publishing Group and the Editor of the Health Education Journal.

We would also like to thank the pharmacy personnel and their customers who participated in this study, and the Chief Scientist Office, Scottish Office Home and Health Department for funding our work.

References

Altman D G (1996). Better reporting of randomised controlled trials: the CONSORT statement. *BMJ* 313: 570–71.

Amos A, Hillhouse A (1992). *Tobacco use in Scotland: a review of literature and research*. Scotland: University of Edinburgh/ASH.

Anonymous (1993). Practice checklist: nicotine replacement therapy. *Pharm J* 255: 291.

Anonymous (1994). Advising on how to stop smoking: guidelines on smoking cessation advice in the pharmacy. *Pharm J* 252: 816.

Ashworth P (1997). Breakthrough or bandwagon? Are interventions tailored to Stage of Change more effective than non-staged interventions? *Health Ed J* 56: 166–74.

Baker T L (1994). *Doing social research*, 2nd edn. New York: McGraw-Hill.

Berbatis C (1991). The pharmacist's involvement in smoking cessation and the use of Nicorette. *Pharm J* 247: 212–14.

Bond C M, Bradley C (1996). The interface between the community pharmacist and patients. *BMJ* 312: 758–60.

Campbell D T, Stanley J C (1963). *Experimental and quasi-experimental design for research*. Chicago: Rand McNally.

Carstairs V, Morris R (1991). *Deprivation and Health in Scotland*. Aberdeen: Aberdeen University Press.

Collett D (1991). *Modelling binary data*. London: Chapman and Hall.

Dixon W J (1993). *BMDP statistical software manual*. Berkeley: University of California Press.

Doll R, Peto R, Wheatley K, *et al.* (1994). Mortality in relation to smoking: 40 years' observations on male British doctors. *BMJ* 309: 901–11.

Donaldson C, Hundley V, Mapp T (1995). *Willingness to pay: a new method for measuring patients' preferences?* HERU Discussion Paper 03/95. University of Aberdeen.

Downie R S, Fyfe C, Tannahill A (1990). *Health Promotion: models and values*. Oxford: Oxford University Press.

Evans D, Moclair A (1994). Vocational qualifications for pharmacy support staff. *Pharm J* 252: 631.

Farmer R, Miller D (1994). *Lecture notes on epidemiology and public health medicine*, 3rd edn. Oxford: Blackwell Scientific Publications.

Flint JF (1995). Planning and recording continuing professional development. *Pharm J* 254: 453.

Genstat 5 Committee (1993). *Genstat 5 reference manual*. Oxford: Clarendon Press.

Goldberg D N, Hoffman A M, Farinha M F, *et al.* (1994). Physician delivery of smoking cessation advice based on the stages-of-change model. *Am J Prev Med* 10(5): 267–74.

Hassell K, Harris J, Rogers A, *et al.* (1996). *The role and contribution of pharmacy in primary care*. Manchester: National Primary Care Research and Development Centre.

Health Education Board for Scotland (1995). *Towards a non-smoking Scotland: a national strategy*. Edinburgh: Health Education Board for Scotland.

Heatherton T F, Kozlowski L T, Frecker R C, *et al.* (1991). The Fagerstrom test for nicotine dependence: a revision of the Fagerstrom tolerance questionnaire. *Br J Addiction* 86: 1119–27.

Institute of Pharmacy Management International (1991). Conference report: market research in community pharmacy. *Pharm J* 247: 612–13.

Jepson M, Jesson J, Kendall H, et al. (1991). Consumer expectations of community pharmaceutical services. London: Department of Health.

Lennox A S, Taylor R J (1994). Factors associated with outcome in unaided smoking cessation, and a comparison of those who have never tried to stop with those who have. Br J Gen Pract 44: 245–50.

Lennox A S, Bain N, Groves J, et al. (1996). The cost-effectiveness of brief training for the primary healthcare team in facilitating smoking behaviour change. Report to the Scottish Office Home and Health Department.

Mant D, Fowler G (1993). Effectiveness of a nicotine patch in helping people stop smoking: results of a randomised trial in general practice. BMJ 306: 1304–8.

Naidoo J, Wills J (1994). Health promotion: foundations for practice. London: Bailliere Tindall.

Nathan A (1995). A non-prescription medicines formulary. Pharm J 255: 547–51.

National Heart Forum (1995). Preventing coronary heart disease in primary care. The way forward. London: HMSO.

Prochaska J O, DiClemente C C (1983). Stages and processes of self change of smoking: toward an integrative model of change. J Consult Clin Psychol 51(3): 390–95.

Prochaska J O, Goldstein M G (1991). Process of Smoking Cessation: implications for clinicians. Clin Chest Med 12(4): 727–35.

Rollnick S, Kinnersley P, Stott N (1993). Methods of helping patients with behaviour change. BMJ 307: 188–90.

Royal Pharmaceutical Society of Great Britain (1995). Pharmacy in a new age: developing a new strategy for the future of pharmacy. London: Royal Pharmaceutical Society of Great Britain.

Royal Pharmaceutical Society of Great Britain (1996). Pharmacy in a new age: the new horizon. London: Royal Pharmaceutical Society of Great Britain.

Russell I T (1984). Clinical trials and evaluation of surgical procedures. Surgery 196–99.

Russell I T, Grimshaw J M (1992). The effectiveness of referral guidelines: a review of the methods and findings of published evaluations. In: Roland M, Coulter A, eds. Hospital referrals. Oxford: Oxford University Press.

Scottish Office (1992). Scotland's Health: a challenge to us all. Edinburgh: HMSO.

Secretary of State for Health (1992). The Health of the Nation: a strategy for health in England. CM 1986. London: HMSO.

Secretary of State for Health (1998). Smoking Kills: a White Paper on tobacco. CM 4177. London: HMSO.

Sharp L K (1985). Prussic Acid, Patients and Professors. Pharm J 235: 821–22.

Silagy C, Lancaster T, Fowler G, et al. (1997). Meta-analysis: Training health care professionals to provide smoking cessation interventions only slightly increases smoking cessation. Evidence-Based Med 2(2): 48.

Sinclair H K (1997). Community pharmacy and smoking cessation: training in behaviour change. PhD Thesis; University of Aberdeen.

Sinclair H K, Bond C M, Lennox A S, et al. (1995). Nicotine Replacement Therapies: smoking cessation outcomes in a community pharmacy setting in Scotland. Tob Control 4: 338–43.

Sinclair H K, Bond C M, Lennox A S, et al. (1997). An evaluation of a training workshop for pharmacists based on the Stages of Change model of smoking cessation. *Health Ed J* 56: 296–312.

Sinclair H K, Bond C M, Lennox A S, *et al.* (1998a). Knowledge of and Attitudes to Smoking Cessation: the effect of stage of change training for community pharmacy staff. *Health Bull* 56(1): 526–39.

Sinclair H K, Bond C M, Lennox A S, *et al.* (1998b). Training pharmacists and pharmacy assistants in the stage-of-change model of smoking cessation: A randomised controlled trial in Scotland. *Tob Control* 7: 253–61.

Sinclair H K, Bond C M, Lennox A S (1999a). The longterm learning effect of training in stage of change for smoking cessation: a three year follow up of community pharmacy staff's knowledge and attitudes. *Int J Pharm Pract* 7: 1–11.

Sinclair H K, Silcock J, Bond C M, *et al.* (1999b). The cost-effectiveness of intensive pharmaceutical intervention in assisting people to stop smoking. *Int J Pharm Pract* 7: 107–12.

Smith F J (1992). Community Pharmacists and Health Promotion: a study of consultations between pharmacists and clients. *Health Promotion International* 7: 249–55.

SPSS for Windows 6.1.3 [computer software] (1995). Chicago, IL: SPSS Inc.

Stott N C H, Rollnick S, Rees M R, *et al.* (1995). Innovation in clinical method: diabetes care and negotiating skills. *Fam Pract* 12: 413–18.

Sutherland G, Stapleton J A, Russell M A, *et al.* (1992). Randomised controlled trial of nasal nicotine spray in smoking cessation. *Lancet* 340: 324–29.

Tang J L, Law M, Wald N (1994). How effective is nicotine replacement therapy in helping people to stop smoking? *BMJ* 308: 21–6.

Vallis J (1994). *Lay people's expectations of community pharmacies.* Vienna: European Society of Medical Sociology Conference.

van Teijlingen E R, Friend J A R, Twine F E (1995). Problems of Evaluation: lessons from a Smokebusters Campaign. *Health Ed J* 54(3): 357–66.

Velicer W F, Prochaska J O, Rossi J S, *et al.* (1992). Asesssing outcome in smoking cessation studies. *Psychol Bull* 111: 23–41.

WHO (1984). 1985 Health Promotion: a WHO Discussion Document on the Concepts and Principles. Copenhagen: World Health Organization.

WHO (1991). 1991 Epidemiology: tobacco attributable mortality, global estimates and projections. *Tobacco Alert.*

Williamson V K, Winn S, Livingstone C R, *et al.* (1992). Public views on an extended role for community pharmacy. *Int J Pharm Pract* 1: 223–9.

9

Health promotion (II): services to drug misusers

Catriona Matheson

Introduction

A harm reduction strategy for tackling drug misuse

A harm reduction approach to drug misuse aims to reduce the individual and social harm associated with the use of illicit drugs. At an individual level, harm reduction aims to prevent the spread of blood-borne diseases through the sharing of injecting equipment and to reduce the incidence of injecting related ill-health such as abscesses, ulcers and gangrene by encouraging safer injecting practices and/or encouraging a shift to non-injecting drug use. At a social level, harm reduction aims to reduce the spread of blood-borne diseases in the non-drug using population and to reduce drug-related crime. The policy of harm reduction was precipitated by the threat to public health of HIV/AIDS in the late 1980s. More recently, additional benefits of reduced spread of other blood-borne diseases such as hepatitis, have been increasingly stated.

Harm reduction in the UK now encompasses the practice of substitute prescribing, that is, the prescribing of Controlled Drugs as a substitute for illicitly obtained drugs, for example, the prescribing of methadone, an opioid, to those using illicit opiates. In short, substitute prescribing aims to shift to non-injecting drug use and removes the need to obtain drugs illegally, thus reducing crime. The management of substitute prescribing in the community setting is the subject of debate at a policy level, since there are concerns that prescribed drugs can be 'leaked' onto the illicit market. In response to this concern, some prescribers require prescriptions to be dispensed daily by the pharmacist and consumed on the pharmacy premises under the supervision of the community pharmacist. This is commonly known as supervised methadone consumption or supervised self-administration of methadone.

The pharmacy profession's perspective

Prior to the harm reduction philosophy the pharmacy profession had a role in preventing drug misuse which resulted in a form of policing of drug misuser activities. For example, until 1986 it was an offence to sell or provide injecting equipment under section 9a of the Misuse of Drugs Act 1971. Therefore, the philosophy of harm reduction was in conflict with the traditional role of the community pharmacist. However, pharmacy's professional body, the Royal Pharmaceutical Society of Great Britain (RPSGB), responded to the challenge of the threat of HIV/AIDS and an amendment to the Misuse of Drugs Act, The Drug Trafficking Offences Act 1986, supported the sale of injecting equipment under certain circumstances.

The management of drug misuse at a societal and individual level is a controversial issue. Policy changes may dictate the expected behaviour of health professionals without explaining the theoretical basis of these policy changes. The introduction of a harm reduction policy resulted in an almost overnight change in the management of drug misusers. Pharmacists had greatly increased contact with drug misusers through their role in dispensing substitute drugs and providing injecting equipment. However, the cultural shift in attitudes to support this change is much slower. The issues are:

- Is the harm reduction policy being implemented as evident by the distribution of services?
- Are pharmacists motivated to provide services for drug misusers because of a harm reduction culture?
- How do attitudes affect the process of service delivery?

Attitudes and behaviour

Attitudes tie together feelings, values and beliefs (Downie *et al.*, 1990). However, the relationship between attitudes and behaviour is not clear cut and requires some consideration. Roedgier *et al.* (1984) defined an attitude as: 'a relatively stable tendency to respond consistently to particular people, objects or situations. ' Downie *et al.* (1990) considered that the use of 'tendency to respond consistently' implied that attitudes do not necessarily determine behaviour. Roedgier *et al.*'s model has only one dimension, i.e. behaviour. Ribeaux and Poppleton's (1978) definition of an attitude: 'a learned predisposition to think, feel and act in a particular way' has three dimensions: thinking (cognitive), feeling (affective) and behaviour. Downie *et al.* (1990) argued that not all three dimensions need to coincide to possess an attitude. For example, a pharmacist may feel sorry for injecting-drug misusers and may believe pharmacists should help reduce the spread of blood-borne diseases, yet will not actually provide a needle/syringe exchange service. There may be opposing factors which pharmacists need to think about and since there is an element of the unknown in introducing a new (to them) service, they do not take that further behavioural step of actually providing the service.

Attitudes of professionals are widely surveyed in the health services, because of the assumption that attitudes determine behaviour. However, behavioural scientists might argue that attitudes are secondary to behaviour, i.e. what people actually do is more important than what they think. Weinman (1987) considered how differences in consultation style were likely to reflect attitudinal differences between doctors concerning their perception of their role, i.e. how their processes of behaviour are affected by their attitude. To summarise the above, people will not always behave according to their expressed attitudes; therefore, attitudes are a predictor of, but not an absolute determinant of, behaviour.

Previous published work in this field

Pharmacists have expressed concerns about the provision of services for drug misusers through correspondence in the *Pharmaceutical Journal* and local surveys. A survey of pharmacists in Greater Glasgow indicated that some pharmacists were worried about the security of stock, staff and other customers when considering whether or not to provide a supervised methadone service (Scott *et al.*, 1994). Similarly, in a Lothian survey, anxiety was revealed about attracting an 'undesirable' client group (Jones *et al.*, 1998).

Concerns have been expressed about the appropriateness of the strategy of harm reduction and the role of the pharmacist. In a letter to the *Pharmaceutical Journal*, Gough (1996) stated that since pharmacists' 'calling was to make sick people better', the emphasis should be on 'encouraging drug misusers to become drug free'. Correspondence in the *Pharmaceutical Journal* regarding negative behaviour by drug misusers reinforces some pharmacists' negative attitudes (Phillips, 1994; Phillips 1996; Green, 1996; Webb, 1998). A survey in two central London Health Authorities found evidence that pharmacists negatively stigmatised drug misusers and this was more likely the longer the respondent had been a community pharmacist (Sheridan and Barber, 1997). A survey of pharmacy students' and pre-registration graduates' attitudes indicated that they were generally positive towards drug misusers but a large proportion (39%) expressed personal fears, indicating feelings of physical vulnerability (Sheridan and Barber, 1993). Negative behaviour by drug misusers is not just a fear resulting from negative attitudes but can be a reality. Indeed, negative behaviour has resulted in the closure of pharmacy needle/syringe exchanges in England (Anonymous, 1996) and in Grampian in Scotland (Bond, personal communication, 1998). In the Lothian survey, 61% of respondents had experienced some problems relating to drug misusers of which violence, abuse and shoplifting were the most common (Jones et al., 1998).

Some pharmacists are more positive and prepared to get involved in services for drug misusers such as supervising methadone consumption and needle/syringe exchange. In Lothian, an area of high prevalence of HIV/AIDS, 29% of survey respondents were involved in a needle/syringe exchange scheme and 79% were currently dispensing substitute drugs (Jones et al., 1998). Forty five per cent of Glasgow pharmacists did or were prepared to supervise methadone consumption (Scott et al., 1994). In West Glamorgan 25 pharmacists supervised methadone consumption (McBride et al., 1993). The survey of pharmacists in two London Health Authorities (n = 285) conducted during 1995 indicated that over half of respondents were involved in dispensing controlled drugs and 13% in needle/syringe exchange (Sheridan and Barber, 1997).

In countries other than the UK, pharmacists are also playing a contributory role in drug misuse. In Mexico pharmacists are involved in community education regarding HIV and sexually transmitted diseases (Pick et al., 1996). In the Netherlands pharmacists provide needle/syringe exchanges in some areas. In parts of the US pharmacists have a role in the care of AIDS patients (Oke, 1995) and as an information source on HIV/AIDS (Binkley et al., 1995). However, the emphasis of pharmacists' involvement in other countries is very much on needle/syringe exchange rather than on substitute prescribing.

Relevance to the extended professional role

There has been much discussion within the pharmacy profession since the publication of the Nuffield Report (Nuffield, 1986) on the appropriateness of providing health services outside the core pharmacy functions (i.e. dispensing and counter prescribing). Drug misuse services may well be considered part of the extended role by individual pharmacists particularly needle/syringe exchange, supervised consumption of methadone and health education of drug misusers. However, other services such as dispensing substitute drugs are core functions.

Although drug misuse services may be considered part of the extended role, there is a definite difference between these services and other extended roles such as cholesterol and blood pressure testing. That is that the need for drug misuse services may be greater in specific communities and this need may not be met by any other healthcare group. In other words there is a very different need and availability profile for drug misuse services.

Research questions and methods

The research questions

Prior to 1995 there had only been small-scale work on the attitudes of pharmacists in the UK, and there had been no published study conducted specifically of Scottish pharmacists at a national level. However, concurrently with the development of the project reported here, a similar study was being developed in England and Wales (Sheridan *et al.*, 1996). This confirms the national gap in evidence which existed at that time. Work on the attitudes of professionals has been conducted with the assumption, although not necessarily explicitly stated, that attitudes affect whether services are provided for drug misusers by general health service providers if they have a 'choice', and the process of care, i.e. how professionals behave. When considering pharmacy specifically there has been no research which links attitudes to the availability of services. Therefore, the first research question is: does the pharmacist's attitude towards drug misusers affect whether or not they provide services to drug misusers?

This leads us to consider the process of service delivery for drug misusers. The process of any service delivery is affected by the attitude of professionals delivering the service (as discussed above). Previous research has focused on the links between pharmacists' attitudes and the structure of services rather than the process of services. This leads us to formulate a second research question: does the pharmacist's attitude towards drug misusers affect the process of service delivery to drug misusers?

Aim and objectives

The aim of the work described in this section is to describe the distribution of drug misuse services in Scottish community pharmacies and investigate the existence and nature of a link between pharmacists' attitudes and the availability and delivery of services.

The specific objectives of the research were to:

- describe the prescribing/dispensing patterns for drug misuse across Scotland as a baseline for further investigation;
- assess the current level of participation of community pharmacists in the provision of services to drug misusers at a national, Scottish level;
- describe the attitudes of community pharmacists towards drug misusers at a national Scottish level; .
- explore if and how pharmacists' attitudes affect whether services are provided and the process of pharmaceutical care;
- assess the attitudes of community pharmacists to an increased involvement in the overall care plan for drug misusers.

Methods

Two complementary methods of data collection were used. This is an accepted methodology in this type of research which requires investigation of issues from different angles, i.e. quantitative and qualitative.

A descriptive survey design was chosen to gain quantitative national data from pharmacists since the aim of the project was to gather baseline data on current attitudes and practice. As it was desirable to get absolute figures for some variables (i.e. the total number of people in Scotland prescribed methadone), the whole community pharmacy population was surveyed. As this was a large population, covering a wide geographical area, a survey using a structured questionnaire was the most cost-effective method (Moser and Kalton, 1986). Furthermore, access to the sampling frame was easy as all community pharmacies are registered and each health board has a current list of pharmacies in that area.

In addition to quantitative data collection, it was desirable to collect in-depth information to provide insight into pharmacists' motivation and attitudes towards providing services for drug misusers. Therefore, a qualitative approach was considered most appropriate (Bryman, 1993). The method of choice was interviewing which can be conducted face-to-face with individuals, by telephone with individuals or in groups (Moser and Kalton, 1986).

Given that the study covered the whole of Scotland, the logistics and resource implications of travelling to conduct face-to-face interviews was considered undesirable. From previous experience, pharmacists have difficulty keeping to specific times because they are usually working in isolation and have to manage issues as they arise. It is not always possible to predict busy times in a pharmacy, so an interviewer could spend a lot of time waiting for the pharmacist to become available.

Therefore, an interviewing schedule could easily overrun. Face-to-face interviews could have been conducted out of work hours. However, the time required for this method would again be severely limiting because only one interview could be conducted per evening due to the geographical spread of interviewees. In addition, if interviews were conducted in pharmacists' homes this may inhibit participation because it is more invasive.

Group interviews or focus groups were not considered appropriate for two reasons. First, an objective of the interviews was to explore attitudes in detail and, if attitudes varied considerably within a group, individuals may be inhibited from revealing their true beliefs. Secondly, organising focus groups to be held in a different part of the country from the researcher's base could pose logistical problems similar to those described above for face-to-face interviews.

Telephone interviews were considered the most appropriate method in this instance. The advantage of a telephone interview is that if the time is inconvenient then the researcher can phone back. Pharmacists were believed to be comfortable communicating by telephone as much of their daily communication is conducted by phone with general practitioners, receptionists, other pharmacists and wholesalers.

The study

National population survey

Questionnaire development and administration

Before compiling the questionnaire, face-to-face, content setting interviews were carried out with eight pharmacists in Grampian and Tayside. These locations were used because they included a range of pharmacy locations (i.e. rural, urban, surburban and city), and patterns of drug misuse (Information and Statistics Division (ISD), 1995) and were readily accessibly for the researcher. A semi-structured interview schedule covered the three broad topic areas of:

- general issues of drug misuse;
- provision of services to drug misusers;
- the pharmacist's role.

These broad headings allowed pharmacists to discuss issues that they felt important.

Following these content-setting interviews, a draft questionnaire was compiled to include:

- demographic information;
- details of current involvement with drug misusers;
- levels of training in this topic area;
- attitudes towards drug misusers;
- willingness to take part in a follow-up telephone interview.

A combination of closed and open questions was used to gain factual information. Open-ended questions were kept to a minimum to keep the questionnaire as simple to complete as possible (Oppenheim, 1992) and open-ended questions were only used to give further details of information given in a closed question.

Demographic information regarding the individual and the pharmacy, past and present levels of involvement with drug misusers and information on past and present training experience were included. Attitudes were surveyed using a series of statements compiled on topics raised in content-setting interviews. Attitudes are complex and may incorporate several dimensions which cannot be covered with a single question (Oppenheim, 1992). Therefore, it was necessary to use a scaling approach, in which individual statements were devised to measure different dimensions. Each statement contributed equally to the attitude scale. It was important to make the statements as meaningful as possible so that pharmacists could relate to statements. A five-point Likert scale, from 'strongly agree' to 'strongly disagree', was used to grade respondents' levels of agreement with each statement (Oppenheim, 1992). Both positive and negative statements were incorporated in the scale. Four questions were reversed and both the positive and negative statements incorporated in the scale, as a measure of internal consistency. Statements covered four broad areas:

- attitudes to drug misusers;
- attitudes to the role of the pharmacist;
- belief in the service i.e. belief in the principles of harm reduction;
- finance.

Statements were arranged randomly to ensure topics were mixed. In addition, it was checked that reversed versions of a statement were not next to each other. This was in order to allow statements to be considered in isolation.

The questionnaire was piloted in a sample of 51 pharmacists randomly selected (using a statistical package) from the population of 1142 pharmacies in Scotland. A covering letter was included, explaining the purpose of the questionnaire. Data from the pilot survey were entered into a database and analysed using basic descriptive statistics.

Following the pilot some minor changes were made to the questionnaire. Those pharmacies included in the pilot were excluded from the main survey to reduce the possibility of 'survey fatigue' which may result in a poor response and thus less accurate data. In addition, responding to the pilot questionnaire may have raised awareness of the issues covered and so the population response may have changed. For individual questions that had not been changed the responses were aggregated with those of the main sample.

A questionnaire, covering letter and reply-paid envelope were sent to pharmacy managers in the remaining 1091 pharmacies in Scotland. The population of pharmacies, rather than a sample was used because the total number of pharmacies in Scotland is not so large as to have enormous resource implications. Surveying the whole population also negates any problems of sampling error or random error in subsequent statistical analysis.

The questionnaire was addressed to the pharmacy manager and the covering letter emphasised that the questionnaire should be completed by the pharmacist who manages the pharmacy on a day-to-day basis. This was to make clear that the questionnaire was aimed at the pharmacist who was most likely to be involved with drug misusers. In most independent pharmacies there is only one pharmacist but in larger pharmacies there may be a management structure or there may be a pharmacy owner who does not actually work in that pharmacy and therefore may not be very familiar with the details of that pharmacy. Clearly defining who should complete the questionnaire should have increased the reliability of the questionnaire.

A reply-paid postcard was enclosed and respondents were requested to post it separately but at the same time as returning the questionnaire. This allowed questionnaires to be anonymous whilst allowing non-responders to be identified. Two reminders were sent to non-responders. It was emphasised that the questionnaire was both confidential and anonymous to ensure that respondents could be honest without fear of reprisal. This was intended to enable a good response rate (Moser and Kalton, 1986).

A database was set up, Statistical Package for Social Scientist, 'SPSS for Windows' (SPSS, 1996), and data entry was performed by an administrative assistant. Data entry was checked by the researcher for errors in 44 questionnaires (1 in 20 sample), selected by the author by randomly picking from the store of returned questionnaires. Few errors were identified indicating accurate data entry.

Analysis of questionnaire data

Attitude scale

Assessment of range of responses and plotting of scores for statistical normality First, the frequency of responses to each statement was assessed to determine whether there was a spread of opinion, as would be expected in a normal population. Secondly, a total score was calculated for each respondent by reversing positive statements then totalling the score for each statement (−2 strongly agree to +2 for strongly disagree). Total scores were plotted for each respondent and the 'normality' of the distribution considered.

Reliability of attitude scale Reliability is the extent to which a measure (the attitude scale) produces the same measurement in the same individual at different points in time. It was not appropriate to re-test the scale (test – re-test reliability) in the same population because this could produce resistance (survey fatigue) in the population (Oppenheim, 1992). Instead, reliability was assessed through internal consistency that is, the extent to which similar items (attitude statements) gave consistent responses (Oppenheim, 1992). This was assessed in two ways: first by comparison of reversed statements to determine if the responses to these statements were consistent with each other; secondly, by determining the Cronbach alpha value, that is the overall correlation between items (in this case statements) within the scale.

Validity of attitude scale Construct validity was assessed by considering whether the responses to individual statements are consistent with the theoretical framework (Oppenheim, 1992). For example, those respondents who run a pharmacy-based needle/syringe exchange might be expected to agree to the statement 'I believe community pharmacy is an appropriate place for a needle/syringe exchange'.

Demography, current practice (behavioural) and training data

Comparison of means T-tests and one way analysis of variances (least significant difference test) were used to compare means of two or more categories as applicable. These parametric tests were the most appropriate because a plot of attitude scores had a normal distribution. Results were considered significant at the 95% confidence level (i.e. $p < 0.05$).

Tests for association Chi-square tests were used to test for association between categories of ordinal variables. Pearson's correlation coefficient was calculated to indicate association between continuous variables.

Telephone interviews with pharmacists

Interview schedule development and administration

Telephone interviews were piloted in a sub-sample of 12 pharmacists identified as having a range of attitude, involvement and location, from those volunteering in the questionnaire. This enabled planning and timetabling of the main interview topic guide. The pilot topic guide included views on:

- supplying injecting equipment (selling and exchanging);
- dispensing to drug misusers (methadone and other drugs);
- attitudes to drug misusers;
- behaviour of drug misusers and effect on other business.

These topics were covered because there was a need to gain more in-depth information than was possible in the questionnaire.

Sixty-five pharmacists were selected for the main interviews, from those volunteering in the national survey questionnaire described earlier. The target was to interview 50 respondents and then re-assess if further interviews were necessary, for example, if new ideas and themes were still emerging. Sixty-five was estimated to be sufficient to take account of possible difficulties in actually contacting interviewees and conducting interviews.

Interviewees were selected to represent a range of experience, attitude, health board area, location of pharmacy (rural/urban/city centre) and type of pharmacy (i.e. single outlet, small or large multiple or health centre). The primary selection criteria were (i) health board area, (ii) level of involvement, and (iii) attitude. Level of involvement was scored according to the number of methadone clients detailed in the questionnaire. Attitude was scored according to their total attitude score. Attitude and involvement were then plotted in tabular form. Secondary criteria were then applied, i.e. type of pharmacy and pharmacy location, by scoring and underlining the respondents code in coloured pen. This plotting exercise allowed a visual representation of the characteristics of those volunteering for interview, which facilitated the selection of interviewees to ensure the range of criteria was covered.

This sampling procedure could be considered as a variation of purposive sampling, in which interviewees were selected to account for factors thought to affect views and relevant to the research questions (Mason, 1996). For example, this study was interested in whether attitudes and views were affected by the location of the pharmacy, attitude of the pharmacists and level of experience (involvement) with drug misusers. Interviewees were therefore sampled to account for the range of these factors as described above.

Interviews were conducted with 45 of those selected. The remaining 20 were unavailable because they had either moved pharmacy, retired, were on holiday or had insufficient time when contacted. It was not felt necessary to select further interviewees from the original sample because after completing 45 interviews no new themes or ideas were emerging. All interviews were tape recorded with the permission of the interviewee.

In addition to the four topics identified for the pilot interviews, the final topic guide included training, misuse of over-the-counter drugs and health promotion. These were added because these topics arose during pilot interviews. Rather than the 'behaviour of drug misusers' and the 'effect on business' it was considered more appropriate to cover under the 'relationship with drug misusers'. This terminology was felt to be less leading, to be comprehensive and positive. The final topic guide included:

- supplying injecting equipment (selling and exchanging);
- dispensing to drug misusers (methadone and other drugs);
- attitudes to drug misusers;
- health promotion advice;
- relationships with drug misusers;
- training;
- misuse of over-the-counter drugs.

All telephone interviews were tape recorded after obtaining the verbal permission of the interviewee. No interviewees declined to have the interview recorded.

Interviews were fully transcribed. Pilot interview data were not included in the analysis because there had been considerable changes to the topic guide. An inductive approach was used to devise a coding format in which recurring themes were noted and when these arose in subsequent interview transcripts a code representing that theme was attached to the text. Coded comments were placed in a table which noted the 'theme', the topic, the interviewee's reference number and attitude scores. All interviews were stored in one large data file which could be sorted according to variable, i.e. theme, topic, attitude or level of involvement. A sample is shown in Table 9.1.

Table 9.1 Example of coding and data management of pharmacist telephone interview data

Ref	Attitude	Involvement	Topic	Theme (code)	Comment	Sub-theme
187	–	M	D2	Mot	It's part of your professional duty is how I see it. I wouldn't refuse to do it.	To provide

Key: – attitude = score < zero, M = medium, D2 = methadone dispensing, Mot = motivation.

Analysis of telephone interview data

Qualitative content analysis was used for analysing data (Morgan, 1993). All comments on a related code (theme) were sorted and analysed together in a new data file. Within this file, comments were subdivided according to topic. For example, for the code 'motivation', all comments were then grouped according to 'needle/syringe exchange', 'selling needles', 'dispensing drugs' 'dispensing methadone' or 'training'.

Coded comments could then be further sorted according to positive or negative attitude and level of involvement (high, medium or low). All comments on a related code and theme could then be studied and the range of opinion expressed (Morgan, 1993) whilst taking into account the attitude and level of involvement of the individual making the comment.

To check the reliability of the data obtained through telephone interviews a copy of the transcript was sent to one in five interviewees selected at random by a statistician using a random number table. A letter accompanied the transcript which stated that if they did not feel the interview reflected their true views they should contact the researcher. No contact was made, indicating they were satisfied with the expression of their views.

Research findings

Response and demography

A response rate of 79.1% (n = 864) was achieved. The number of respondents including the pilot was 902. An almost equal number of male and female pharmacists responded (50.8% male, 47.9% female). A higher proportion of respondents was based in urban pharmacies

(48.6% compared to 21.4% rural and 28.1% city centre). There was a fairly even spread of respondents from different types of pharmacy (35.2% single outlets, 28.4% small multiples, 29.1% large multiples and 2.3% health centre). Over half of respondents had sole decision-making responsibility, a third shared decision making with another person and just 11.5% of respondents had no such responsibility. The average age was 39.9 years (standard deviation (SD) 11.6).

The mean attitude score was 4.2 (SD 16.3) and a plot of attitude score indicated a normal distribution as shown in Figure 9.1. A one-way analysis of variance indicated that there was a significant difference between the mean attitude score in different health boards (Table 9.2). The mean attitude score for a large metropolitan health board area, area eight (9.7, SD 15.95) was significantly higher than area seven, a mixed city/rural area (0.3, SD 17.28) and area five, a mixed urban/rural area (−0.8, SD 15.0), (p < 0.000 1). Although the mean attitude scores for areas four and ten appear higher, these are not significant due to the smaller numbers of respondents.

A one-way analysis of variance indicated there was a significant difference in attitude score according to the pharmacy location. A least significant difference test indicated that city centre pharmacists had a

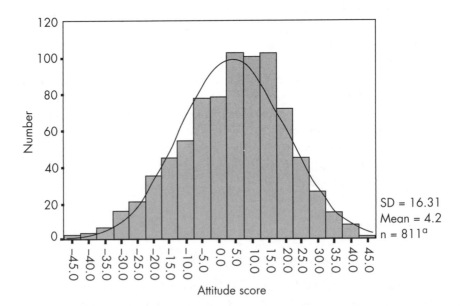

Figure 9.1 Histogram of the attitude scores of the pharmacist population. [a]Only 811 respondents answered all 27 attitude statements

Table 9.2 Mean attitude score of respondents by Health Board area and type

Health Board	Health Board type	Respondents	Mean score (SD)
1	urban/rural	60	3.73 (16.03)
2	urban/rural	56	1.11 (15.41)
3	rural	20	1.75 (17.78)
4	urban/rural	26	11.15 (13.09)
5	urban/rural	53	−0.81 (15.00)
6	urban	50	5.04 (15.47)
7	city/urban/rural	106	0.30 (17.28)
8	city/suburban	143	9.70 (15.95)
9	urban/rural	31	5.81 (16.42)
10	rural	7	11.86 (9.65)
11	urban/rural	68	1.97 (15.15)
12	city/urban/rural	118	4.43 (16.75)
13	city/urban/rural	66	3.85 (16.81)

significantly higher attitude score (6.5, SD 17.3) than both urban (3.4, SD 16.0) and rural (3.1, SD 15.9), ($p = 0.043$). A t-test indicated there was no significant difference in mean attitude score between male, (4.6, SD 17.5) and female pharmacists (3.8, 15.1), ($p = 0.49$). There was no significant difference in mean attitude score according to whether the respondent was based in a single outlet (3.1, SD 18.0), a small multiple (3.9, SD 14.8), a large multiple (5.2, SD 15.7) or a health centre (10.8, SD 10.8), ($p = 0.15$). There was no significant correlation between attitude score and either age (Pearson's Correlation Coefficient, $r = 0.15$) or number of years experience (Pearson's Correlation Coefficient, $r = 0.15$).

Needle/syringe exchange services

Only 8.6% of respondents provided a needle/syringe exchange service. Reasons given in an open-ended question, for not providing this service were that:

- there was no demand in the area;
- another pharmacy provided this service;
- pharmacies were not considered an appropriate place, and the service should be provided by a clinic.

When asked, 37.5% of respondents currently sold needles/syringes. A further 17.3% were prepared to but had no demand, leaving a considerable proportion (45.1%) who were not prepared to sell needles/

syringes. The breakdown by health board is shown in Table 9.3. A higher proportion of respondents in areas six and seven were currently selling needles compared to other areas. Pharmacists in area eight were the least likely to sell needles/syringes with 64.9% being unwilling to do so. A t-test indicated that those providing a needle/syringe exchange service have significantly higher attitude scores than those who do not (p < 0.000 1) (see Table 9.4).

Substitute drug dispensing services

Of all respondents, 61% dispensed drugs for the management of drug misuse. Methadone was the most frequently dispensed drug (76.8%), followed by diazepam (59.5%), dihydrocodeine (43.3%) and temazepam (40.9%). Of all respondents, 54.6% dispensed methadone at the time of the survey with a wide variation by health board area ranging from 75.3% to 26.2%. The majority of methadone prescribing is managed on prescriptions from general practice although this varies according to health board area. Sixty-five percent of prescribing is on a daily basis. There is some variation in dispensing interval according to health board ranging from 89.1% on a daily basis compared to just 16.7% (Table 9.5).

Table 9.3 Willingness to sell needles/syringes by Health Board (including pilot, n = 881)

Health Board	No. respondents	Yes, currently do No. (%)	Yes, no demand No. (%)	No No. (%)
1	68	9 (13.2)	22 (32.3)	37 (54.4)
2	74	11 (14.9)	32 (43.2)	31 (41.9)
3	22	1 (4.5)	13 (59.1)	8 (36.4)
4	27	2 (7.4)	13 (48.1)	12 (44.4)
5	60	6 (10.0)	25 (41.7)	29 (48.3)
6	51	17 (33.3)	19 (37.2)	15 (29.4)
7	111	35 (31.5)	34 (30.6)	42 (37.8)
8	154	22 (14.9)	32 (20.8)	100 (64.9)
9	34	2 (5.9)	20 (58.8)	12 (35.3)
10	8	0 (0.0)	5 (62.5)	3 (37.5)
11	76	7 (9.2)	34 (44.7)	35 (46.1)
12	123	26 (21.1)	50 (40.6)	47 (38.2)
13	73	16 (21.9)	31 (42.5)	26 (35.6)
Total	881	154 (17.5)	330 (37.5)	397 (45.1)

Table 9.4 Mean attitude score versus service provision. (Modified with permission from Matheson *et al.*, 1999b.)

Service provided	Yes mean score (SD)	No mean score (SD)	Don't know mean score	Significant difference
1 Needle/syringe exchange	15.7 (14.8)	3.1 (16.0)	NR	S (p < 0.001)
2 Methadone dispensing	6.5 (16.0)	0.75 (16.4)	NR	S (p < 0.001)
3 Supervising methadone consumption	12.7 (13.8)	5.9 (15.7)	NR	S (p < 0.001)
4 Prepared to supervise methadone	14.5 (11.7)	−6.8 (12.6)	10.1 (11.8)	S (p < 0.001)

Table 9.5 Daily methadone prescribing by Health Board and source of prescription. (Modified from Matheson *et al.*, 1999a.)

Health Board	GP10 Prescriptions % daily	Hospital/clinic % daily	Overall % daily	No. methadone users on a supervised daily dose (%)
1	75.6	87.0	79.8	13 (10.4)
2	37.8	48.7	45.3	4 (3.4)
3	16.7	0	16.7	0 (0)
4	14.3	24.5	23.9	13 (11.4)
5	59.3	39.4	57.1	0 (0)
6	39.2	39.4	39.3	3 (2.4)
7	48.8	70.2	54.1	68 (19.3)
8	89.5	86.7	89.1	994 (69.7)
9	69.2	66.7	67.9	1 (3.6)
10	50.0	0	50.0	10 (17.2)
11	66.1	75.0	66.7	8 (1.3)
12	31.7	40.0	33.3	1 (0.3)
13	46.2	75.7	58.0	0 (0)
Total	66.8	61.8	65.6	1115 (32.9)

Pharmacy supervision of methadone consumption by the drug misuser varied considerably across health boards (69.7%–0%) (Table 9.5). Correspondingly, the involvement of pharmacies in providing a supervised methadone consumption service varies (Table 9.6) ranging from 65.4% of pharmacies to 0%.

Amongst those not currently providing a 'supervision' service, willingness to supervise methadone consumption also varied considerably, ranging from 31.2% to 2.7% (Table 9.6). Those respondents who

Table 9.6 Pharmacy supervision of methadone consumption by Health Board. (Modified from Matheson *et al.*, 1999a.)

Health Board	No. respondents (including pilot)	No. dispensing methadone, including pilot (%)	No. currently supervising methadone, including pilot (%)	No. prepared to supervise methadone but no present demand, including pilot (%)
1	69	37 (53.6)	11 (15.9)	16 (23.2)
2	75	31 (41.3)	5 (6.7)	11 (14.7)
3	22	8 (36.4)	0 (0.0)	3 (13.6)
4	27	14 (51.8)	5 (18.5)	5 (18.5)
5	60	28 (46.7)	2 (3.3)	4 (6.7)
6	52	29 (55.8)	3 (5.2)	10 (19.2)
7	112	59 (52.7)	26 (23.2)	14 (12.5)
8	156	117 (75.0)	102 (65.4)	9 (5.8)
9	37	11 (29.7)	1 (2.7)	8 (21.6)
10	5	2 (40.0)	0 (0.0)	0 (0.0)
11	80	21 (26.2)	5 (6.2)	25 (31.2)
12	126	83 (65.9)	9 (7.1)	19 (15.1)
13	73	48 (65.7)	1 (1.4)	2 (2.7)
Total	894	488 (54.6)	170 (19.0)	126 (14.1)

were not prepared to supervise methadone consumption were asked in an open-ended question to identify what would encourage them to supervise methadone consumption. Remuneration/payment was the most frequently mentioned factor (56%) followed by 'nothing' (43.9%), 'if it would prevent selling on the streets' (28.8%) and 'having a private area' (26.5%).

A t-test indicated those who were dispensing methadone at the time of the survey had a significantly higher attitude score than those not dispensing ($p < 0.0001$) (see Table 9.4). There was no significant difference between those who had ever had to withdraw a methadone dispensing service to an individual and those who had not. Those respondents providing a supervised methadone consumption service had significantly higher attitude score than those who were not (t-test, $p < 0.0001$).

Current dispensing and health promotion practice

The provision of health promoting services by pharmacists either in the form of verbal or written information was extremely low for both advice on drug misuse and HIV prevention (Table 9.7). A significant difference was found in the mean attitude score between those who:

- always make up prescriptions in advance compared to never;
- always or sometimes supply leaflets on drug misuse compared to never;
- sometimes supply leaflets on HIV prevention compared to never (see Note 1, p. 207);
- always offer face-to-face advice on drug misuse compared to never;
- always offer face-to-face advice on drug misuse compared to sometimes;
- always or sometimes offer face-to-face advice on HIV prevention compared to never;
- always treat drug misusers the same as other customers compared to sometimes or never.

Further details of the questionnaire survey are reported elsewhere (Matheson *et al.* 1999a; Matheson *et al.*, 1999b).

Summary of main findings from pharmacist interviews

The following is a summary of the main issues identified in the pharmacy interviews. Full details of these have been reported elsewhere (Matheson and Bond, 1999).

- Pharmacists are motivated to provide drug misuse services (i) to help reduce the spread of blood-borne diseases, (ii) because of an awareness of a need for services in the local community and (iii) due to a desire to extend their professional role.
- Barriers to providing services are (i) concerns for the effect on other customers, (ii) anxiety over safety, (iii) concern over the workload and (iv) because remuneration was not believed to be adequate for the workload involved. The suitability of the location and size of the premises was an issue.
- Specific motivation for supervising methadone consumption was to prevent leakage onto the illicit market.
- There were no specific barriers to displaying health promotion leaflets on drug misuse but interviewees had not made a conscious effort to obtain and display such leaflets.
- Pharmacists were inhibited from giving verbal advice and information to drug misusers due to a fear of rejection or confrontation. As a result, verbal advice was largely reactive rather than proactive.
- Some interviewees were uncomfortable with the principles of harm reduction and others did not appear to fully understand it.
- There was concern that funding for methadone prescribing and dispensing was inadequate and new money was required.
- Some pharmacists felt isolated. Communication with other services could be minimal but where good links existed these were considered beneficial and a good source of information.

Table 9.7 Mean attitude score versus details of current practice[a]. (Modified with permission from Matheson et al., 1999b.)

	Always	Mean attitude score	Sometimes	Mean attitude score	Never	Mean attitude score	Significant difference between groups at 95% CI?
	No. (%)		No. (%)		No. (%)		
Lay down ground rules for new person	254 (55.5)	9.61	144 (31.4)	7.33	60 (6.9)	5.84	NS (p = 0.149)
Have a written contract	11 (2.4)	17.33	24 (5.3)	10.13	420 (92.3)	8.05	NS (p = 0.168)
Ask for ID on first visit	121 (26.6)	7.13	146 (32.1)	10.35	188 (41.3)	7.30	NS (p = 0.141)
Ask for ID when collecting supply	66 (14.6)	8.02	146 (32.2)	8.56	241 (53.2)	8.11	NS (p = 0.956)
Make up in advance	238 (52.1)	9.79	145 (31.7)	7.85	74 (16.2)	4.82	S (p = 0.0498)
Provide measures to take away	107 (23.6)	9.20	259 (57.0)	8.64	88 (19)	6.69	NS (p = 0.513)
Supply information leaflets on drug misuse	12 (2.6)	19.45	162 (35.4)	14.04	283 (61.9)	4.71	S (p = 0.000)
Supply information leaflets on HIV prevention	9 (2)	13.89	172 (37.8)	12.91	274 (60.2)	5.41	S (p = 0.000)
Offer face-to-face advice on drug misuse	25 (5.5)	20.14	209 (45.9)	13.87	221 (48.6)	2.05	S (p = 0.000)
Offer face-to-face advice on HIV prevention	12 (2.6)	23.00	127 (28.0)	17.72	315 (69.6)	4.19	S (p = 0.000)
Treat drug users the same as other customers	342 (75.2)	10.76	92 (20.2)	1.17	21 (4.6)	0.48	S (p = 0.000)

Key: NS = Not Significant, S = Significant
[a]The denominator varies for each question because missing values were not included in this analysis

Implications of findings for pharmacy practice

The process of pharmaceutical care: attitudes and practice

Demographic factors had an effect on attitude, with several variables displaying statistical associations. Attitudes varied according to health board region. Regional differences may be related to regional differences in character, for example pharmacists in one part of the country may be more outgoing than those in another part of the country. It may be partly linked to the level of involvement with drug misusers since the area with the second highest mean attitude score also had the highest level of dispensing involvement. However, this area was also remunerated for supervising methadone consumption while other areas were not at the time of the survey. It is possible that remuneration would not only encourage more pharmacists to provide the service but may even be linked to a change in attitude, perhaps because they feel more valued or feel they have had a positive professional endorsement of this service from the local health board.

Pharmacists in city centre pharmacies had significantly more positive attitudes and, again, this may be linked to their level of involvement with drug misusers compared to rural or even urban pharmacies. From these results it is not possible to prove definitively whether those with more positive attitudes are more likely to become involved or whether their attitudes have changed as a result of their involvement. Interview data suggested both mechanisms operate, since those providing a needle/syringe exchange service, and who have thereby opted into this service, have more positive attitudes. In addition, a few interviewees revealed they had been wary about drug misusers but, with experience, found their concerns were unfounded.

Survey data indicated one-off adverse events ('antisocial' behaviour) did not appear to affect a pharmacist's attitude. However, correspondence in the literature (Anonymous, 1996) indicated that pharmacists were likely to withdraw services following adverse events. The frequency of negative incidents may be important as well as other factors such as the personalities involved and the exact nature of the adverse event(s).

Survey results proved that attitudes were clearly linked to the provision of services whether selling needles/syringes, providing a needle/syringe exchange, dispensing methadone, supervising methadone consumption or providing health promotion services in the form of advice and leaflets to drug misusers. Attitudes towards providing each of these services varied, presumably because ethical or professional concerns and perceived risks vary for each service. For example, only 9% of pharmacists provided a needle/syringe exchange yet this group had a high mean attitude score of 15.7. Nineteen percent currently provided a supervised methadone service, with a mean score of 12.7 and over 50% provided a methadone service with a mean score of 6.5. Results indicated that providing a needle/syringe exchange is limited to the most positive and, from interview findings, the most motivated pharmacists because of the greater perceived risks associated with this service.

Pharmacists have to opt into providing a needle/syringe exchange, whereas all pharmacists are contractually obliged to dispense methadone if requested on prescription. Pharmacists are not contractually obliged to provide a supervised methadone service but do not usually have to formally opt into this service provision as with a needle/syringe exchange. Consequently, some pharmacists may have found themselves providing services they would rather not provide if given a choice. Other reasons for the mean attitude score for methadone dispensing being lower than other services may relate back to the perceived role of a community pharmacist. Pharmacists are familiar with the dispensing role, which is one of their core functions, whereas both needle/syringe exchange and supervising methadone consumption are newer roles.

The delivery of services was related to attitude. Those who did not make up prescriptions in advance had a lower attitude score, perhaps indicating less consideration of the needs of the drug misuser. However, there may be other considerations, such as the security of storing prepared prescriptions and the size of the controlled drugs cabinet. Those who believed that they treated drug misusers the same as other customers had a more positive attitude. Therefore, both the professional services and the personal relationship provided by the pharmacist for drug misusers may be affected by their attitude (Matheson *et al.*, 1999b; Matheson and Bond, 1999).

Service delivery may be affected by the number of clients. For example, some pharmacists may not make up prescriptions in advance because they have fewer methadone clients and therefore more time and/or because they have a negative attitude. Analysis of data on the effect of number of clients was limited, as it was considered outside the remit of the investigation but would be an interesting area of further study.

The evidence of regional differences in the attitudes towards, and treatment of, drug misusers indicates that initiatives aimed at changing attitudes should perhaps be area specific. It may also indicate that attitudes may be different as a result of regional initiatives.

The pharmacist's role in overall care of drug misusers

Many pharmacists were uncomfortable with the principles of methadone maintenance perhaps because, as one interviewee indicated, it goes against the principles by which pharmacists have traditionally been educated, that is that drug misuse is a 'social evil' and pharmacy's role is to police drug misuse. Drug misusers in the past only went into pharmacies for negative reasons, such as to try to obtain injecting equipment (which was illegal at the time), so actually to offer help and encourage such people into pharmacies through prescribing (or needle/syringe exchange) is a role reversal for all but the most recently qualified pharmacists. Despite this discomfort, many interviewees understood the principles of harm reduction and acknowledged, perhaps grudgingly, that community pharmacies were the obvious and easiest way of providing a methadone service at a societal level.

There were still some pharmacists who were unclear about the principles of harm reduction and the rationale for methadone maintenance therapy. They expect doses of methadone to be reduced more rapidly and/or eventual abstinence to be the sole objective. The lack of progress with treatment may have frustrated some pharmacists who, although they thought they understood the principles of harm reduction, could not endorse the principles in practice and did not really believe in it. This may be due to a lack of understanding of the drug misuser's lifestyle and problems. Drug misuse training for pharmacists must not only inform pharmacists of the principles of harm reduction on paper, but also be sufficiently in-depth to understand the drug misusers' perspective.

The communication links with other service providers, particularly those prescribing for drug misuse, could be an area of conflict. Where there were good communication links, pharmacists appeared to feel more positive. These links not only made pharmacists feel more involved, but could also be a source of useful information. Lack of apparent action and feedback from a drug agency when a pharmacist contacts them regarding a client will inhibit pharmacists from future contact. Feedback from agencies and general practitioners following a pharmacist's contact would strengthen links and facilitate communication.

In some cases, more often with general practitioners than other prescribing agencies, pharmacists seemed to be wary of contacting prescribers other than when it was essential. Pharmacists were particularly reticent when it came to prescribing issues and clearly did not like to question the wisdom of prescribing practices with the prescriber, although they had legitimate concerns about specific prescriptions. This may have been because they were unsure of the response or concerned that they may put the prescriber in a difficult position. There is evidence from other areas of pharmacy practice that pharmacists and general practitioners working together can be beneficial and lead to improvements in prescribing practice (Goldstein et al., 1998). If pharmacists were to receive local encouragement at health board level and professional endorsement for this role they may be more proactive in dealing with prescribing queries.

Service planning and professional endorsement of services

These research findings have implications for the future planning of services. Should reluctant pharmacists be 'forced' to provide services to which they are opposed? This question cannot be answered completely without considering the effect of the pharmacist's attitude on the outcome of care. Other research has indicated that negative attitudes are counterproductive, causing distress to the drug misuser and the pharmacist and staff (Matheson, 1998). However, the volume of drug misusers needing pharmacy services must also be considered as some pharmacists are overburdened with the sheer numbers of drug misusers attending their pharmacy. Ideally, the attitudinal barriers of negative pharmacists should be addressed as well as providing incentives to provide services. Encouraging more pharmacists to provide services in this way would spread the workload and keep numbers of clients for each to a manageable level.

A working party was set up by the Royal Pharmaceutical Society of Great Britain to look at the profession's contribution to the prevention of HIV/AIDS, Hepatitis B and C and sexually transmitted diseases (Royal Pharmaceutical Society Working Party, 1997). The working party made ten main recommendations, which were subsequently endorsed by the Council of the Royal Pharmaceutical Society of Great Britain. These recommendations included setting standards for a supervised methadone consumption service and encouraging pharmacists to display leaflets and be more proactive in providing information to drug misusers.

At a worldwide level the World Health Organization (WHO) and the International Pharmaceutical Federation (FIP) issued a joint declaration which recognised pharmacists as 'the most numerous and accessible 'health outlet' for the general public'. Therefore, a set of guiding principles was compiled for pharmacists on the approaches to take, in the fight against HIV/AIDS. These principles included developing training programmes, facilitating communication with other professionals to pool talents and promote a co-ordinated approach, and encouraging pharmacists to become involved in decision making at a national public policy level.

In conclusion, pharmacists are experiencing personal conflict over their professional role. Individual pharmacists have to overcome attitudinal barriers which are often caused by their confusion over what is an appropriate professional role. Pharmacists need to receive professional endorsement to feel more comfortable about providing harm reduction services for drug misusers. Professional endorsement includes the acknowledgement at a national and local level such as support from the Royal Pharmaceutical Society of Great Britain and practice guidance from the Code of Ethics, which would indicate that the services they provide are valued. Consultation with pharmacists in drug misuse service planning, communication from other service providers and direct remuneration for services are indicators of professional endorsement to the pharmacist.

These changes are already starting to occur. Pharmacists are increasingly acknowledged by other professionals and policy makers as being essential to the harm reduction strategy.

Note

1. There may be no significant difference between the 'always' category and 'never' because there were only nine respondents who 'always' supplied leaflets.

Acknowledgements

We would like to thank the Chief Scientist Office, Scottish Office Home and Health Department for funding the project and all the pharmacists who took part. This work was originally published in Addiction (Matheson *et al.*, 1999b) and in Family Practice (Matheson *et al.*, 1999a), and is reproduced with permission.

References

Anonymous (1996). News. Abuse drives pharmacies out of needle scheme. *Pharm J* 257: 341.
Binkley D, Waller L, Potts L, *et al.* (1995). Pharmacists as HIV/AIDS information resources: survey of Alabama pharmacists. *AIDS Educ Prev* 7(5): 455–66.
Bryman A (1993). *Quantity and Quality in Social Research*. London: Routledge.
Downie R S, Fyfe C, Tannahill A (1990). *Health Promotion: models and values*. Oxford: Oxford University Press.

Drug Trafficking Offences Act (1986). London: HMSO.

Gough D R (1996). Needle Exchange: A compromise for the future. *Pharm J* 257: 264.

Green C (1996). Drug abuse: methadone supply. *Pharm J* 257: 307.

Information and Statistics Division, National Health Service in Scotland (1995). Drug Misuse Statistics in Scotland 1995 Bulletin. Edinburgh: ISD Publications.

Jones P, van Teijlingen E, Matheson C, *et al.* (1998). Pharmacists' approach to harm minimisation initiatives associated with problem drug use: the Lothian survey. *Pharm J* 260: 324–27.

Matheson C, Bond C M (1999). Motivations and barriers to community pharmacy services for drug misusers. *IJPP* 7: 256–53.

Matheson C, Bond C M, Hickey (1999a). Prescribing and dispensing for drug misusers: current practice in Scotland. *Fam Pract* 16(4): 375–79.

Matheson C, Bond C M, Mollison J (1999b). Attitudinal factors associated with community pharmacists' involvement in services for drug misusers. *Addiction* 94(9): 1349–59. Published by Carfax, www.tandf.co.uk

McBride A J, Meredith-Smith P, Davies M E (1993). Helping injecting drug users – a role for community pharmacists? *Pharm J* 250: 708–9.

Misuse of Drugs Act (1971). London: HMSO.

Moser C A Kalton G (1986). *Survey methods in social investigation*. Hants: Gower.

Oke T (1995). The role of pharmacists in AIDS care delivery. *Aids Patient Care* April: 75–7.

Oppenheim A N (1992). *Questionnaire design, interviewing and attitude measurement*. London: Pinter.

Phillips J (1994). *Back to Basics*. *Pharm J* 252: 109.

Phillips J (1996). Needle Exchange: Said it all Before! *Pharm J* 257: 392.

Pick S, Reyes J, Alvarez M, *et al.* (1996). AIDS prevention training for pharmacy workers in Mexico City. *AIDS Care* 8(1): 55–69.

Ribeaux S, Poppleton S E (1978). *Psychology and work – an introduction*. London: Macmillan.

Roedigier H L, Rushton J P, Capaldi E D, Paris S G (1984). *Psychology*. Boston: Little Brown.

Scott R T A, Burnett S J, McNulty H (1994). Supervised administration of methadone by pharmacists. *BMJ* 308: 1438.

Sheridan J, Barber N (1993). Pharmacy undergraduates' and pre-registration pharmacists' attitudes towards drug misuse and HIV. *J Soc Admin Pharm* 10: 163–70.

Sheridan J, Barber N (1997). Drug Misuse and HIV Prevention: attitudes and practices of community pharmacists with respect to two London Family Health Services. *Addiction Research* 5(1): 11–21.

Sheridan J, Strang J, Barber N, *et al.* (1996). Role of community pharmacies in relation to HIV prevention and drug misuse: findings from the 1995 national survey in England and Wales. *BMJ* 313: 272–4.

Webb D (1998). Aggravation, expense and ill will. *Pharm J* 260: 486.

Weinman J (1987). An outline of psychology as applied to medicine. Oxford: Butterworth Heinmann.

10

Conclusion: the future for evidence-based pharmacy

Alison Blenkinsopp

Introduction

This final chapter reviews the extent and robustness of the evidence for the range of pharmacists' roles. It also considers the future agenda, in the light of the evidence, for practitioners, researchers and those involved in service development.

Evidence to support the 'Pharmacy in a New Age' (PIANA) strategy

The five key roles identified in PIANA and the supporting evidence presented in this book are summarised in Table 10.1.

Table 10.1 Evidence for the five PIANA key roles

PIANA role	Evidence presented in this book
Management of prescribed medicines	Pharmacist-managed repeat prescribing (Chapter 5)
Management of chronic conditions	Pharmacist-led ulcer management clinics (Chapter 6)
	Hospital at Home (Chapter 7)
Management of minor ailments	Advice-giving in community pharmacy (Chapter 2)
	Guidelines and use of POM to P medicines (Chapter 3)
	Cost-effectiveness of POM to P switches (Chapter 4)
Promotion of healthy lifestyles	Advice on smoking cessation (Chapter 8)
	Attitudes to drug misuse services (Chapter 9)
Advice to other health professionals	

In the analysis that follows, selected key studies from recent literature (1997–99) are used to assess the picture of research evidence for each of the five themes. This is not a systematic review, rather a themed synthesis of evidence from the UK, Europe, US and Australian pharmacy practice research.

Management of prescribed medicines

The development of 'cognitive' services and the move away from a supply-oriented role has long been recognised as a prerequisite for the long-term survival of community pharmacy. The potential for community pharmacists to positively influence treatment from the pharmacy setting has, to some extent, been overlooked in the move to establish pharmacists as advisers at the point of prescribing in primary care, i.e. in general medical practices. As the report of the Royal Pharmaceutical Society's working group on Getting Research Into Practice puts it, there are 'opportunities to monitor progress and to revisit prescribing decisions using the dispensing process as the framework'. However, these are under-utilised, and 'thus the community pharmacist's own practice, and contact with patients, has not been included in initiatives to improve the use and uptake of evidence' (Royal Pharmaceutical Society of Great Britain, 1999). Research findings in this area have been published. A study carried out in Tayside indicated the benefits from a scheme in which community pharmacists managed repeat prescriptions (Dowell *et al.*, 1998). In Chapter 5, Bond described the outcomes of a randomised controlled trial of pharmacist-managed repeat prescribing (or 'repeat dispensing' as it has also been termed) carried out in Grampian. The findings of the study showed that the new service was acceptable to patients and doctors, and that more drug-related problems were identified in the intervention group (Bond *et al.*, 2000). This Scottish study provided further evidence to support the community pharmacist's role in monitoring repeat medication in the pharmacy setting. One of the reasons for this study's importance is that it is one of the first to test a new service in the general setting of community pharmacy rather than among a small number of enthusiasts. Further research is now needed to explain the inter-pharmacy variations in identification of adverse drug reactions and drug-related problems found in the study, and their implications for patient care. Were these, for example, due to differences in detection rates by pharmacists or to variations in prescribing quality?

In the US the Kaiser Permanente/USC programme has shed light on the effects of pharmacists' interventions in the community/primary care setting (McCombs *et al.*, 1998). Their multi-centre pharmacy-based study examined the effects of three models of pharmacist consultation – the 'state' model (legal requirement for pharmacist counselling on all new or changed medications), the 'Kaiser-Permanente, KP' model (targeted counselling at selected 'at risk' patients) and 'usual care'. The findings were complex and indicate that the KP model led to a reduction in hospital admissions and healthcare resource use, and that these potential cost savings were offset by increased pharmacist staff costs. There was also the suggestion that drug costs may have increased as a result of enhanced compliance. The KP programme offers tantalising indications of benefit from pharmacist intervention which now need further research to refine the model.

Trials of medication review by pharmacists in the primary care medical practice setting have shown positive outcomes (Mackie *et al.*, 1999; Granas and Bates, 1999), and a recent review shows that further work is now needed (Tully and Cantrill, 1999). Medication management in non-hospital residential settings is another key area. The randomised controlled trial conducted by Furniss and colleagues was the first in the UK to investigate the effects of pharmacist input in the nursing home setting (Furniss *et al.*, 1998). The study took place in 14 nursing homes and the outcome measures included resident functioning and use of primary and secondary care resources. The findings showed that patients in the intervention group had fewer hospital admissions and that the most frequent recommendation made by the pharmacist was to discontinue medication.

Management of chronic conditions

The practice-based pharmacist's role is also explored in Macgregor's study of pharmacist-based ulcer management clinics in primary care (Chapter 6). The same research team had previously evaluated a pharmacist-led anticoagulant clinic in primary care and shown the service to match the quality and accuracy of that provided by the local hospital as well as being acceptable to patients and more convenient for them (Macgregor *et al.*, 1996). Patients with chronic conditions previously cared for in hospital are increasingly being managed in domiciliary settings. Such patients include the terminally ill, and those requiring ongoing treatment during recovery. The potential input of the pharmacist in caring for these patients is described in another Scottish study reported by Williams in Chapter 7. The generalisability of findings from hospital-trained clinical pharmacists in small single practice studies is as yet unknown. However, the results of studies to date appear promising.

The pharmacist's role in the management of diabetes was studied in the US in primary care clinics serviced by one clinical pharmacist from a hospital setting. Patients were referred to the pharmacist by primary care providers, generally where control was proving difficult. The pharmacist was authorised to initiate insulin treatment and to adjust doses in patients already using insulin. This small study (23 patients) showed that glycaemic control improved in most although only a minority achieved an acceptable level of control (Coast-Senior et al., 1998).

In the US a randomised controlled trial investigated the effects of pharmacist monitoring and intervention on the control of hypertension and management of chronic obstructive pulmonary disease (COPD). The study involved ten pharmacies in the community setting, 98 patients with hypertension and 133 with COPD (Gourley et al., 1998a, b). The outcome measures included patient knowledge, medication compliance, patient satisfaction and quality of life. Blood pressure readings were taken by pharmacists for the patients with hypertension, and COPD patients self-reported on their degree of breathlessness and symptom levels. Patients in the intervention group for hypertension had a significantly greater reduction in blood pressure than the controls. Although trends in the COPD group favoured the intervention group the differences did not reach statistical significance (Solomon et al., 1998).

A controlled trial of the community pharmacist's role in hypertension has recently been completed in the UK (Blenkinsopp et al., 2000). The trial intervention (a brief questioning protocol to structure discussion about the patient's medicines) was designed to be applied in any community pharmacy. The results showed improved blood pressure control, an increase in self-reported adherence and increased patient satisfaction among patients in the intervention group, all of which were statistically significant. The generalisability of these promising findings beyond the pharmacies in the intervention group to the wider community pharmacy setting requires further research.

Management of minor ailments

Smith and colleagues have described the range and incidence of symptoms presented in community pharmacies and the resulting responses (Chapter 2). Their work in assessing the quality and appropriateness of advice in a sub-sample of consultations identified that while advice given was generally sound, weaknesses were identified in some areas. More recently, the work of Bissell and Ward has highlighted the variation between community pharmacies in the way the process of responding to symptoms and to requests for medicine purchases were handled (Bissell *et al.*, 1997; Ward *et al.*, 1998). The same team developed and tested a method to assess the appropriateness of pharmacist's and assistants' consultations with clients about OTC medicines (Bissell *et al.*, 2000). The new method offers the opportunity for futher research.

Similar variation in the type and quality of response to symptoms has also been reported in the US (Lamsam and Kropff, 1998). Their results showed that about one third of recommendations were appropriate and one third were poor. In one in three cases recommendations were made without prior assessment of the patient's problem. The development of clinical guidelines for community pharmacists and their assistants to use when providing advice in response to symptoms goes some way to addressing variations in this aspect of pharmacy (see Chapter 3). Such guidelines, evidence-based, must be continually updated and cover the range of therapeutic areas likely to be most frequently advised on in the community pharmacy setting.

Relatively little attention has been paid to the extent to which community pharmacists' recommendations for-over-the counter medicines are evidence-based. An Australian study sought to identify the factors used by community pharmacists in deciding which ingredient(s) and brand to recommend (Roins, 1998). The authors found that the 'clinical influences' construct explained the highest percentage of variation in choice of ingredient (around 20%). Further research is needed in this area to map influences across different symptom and therapy groups.

Promotion of healthy lifestyles

The randomised controlled trial of the effects of community pharmacist's smoking cessation advice reported by Sinclair (Chapter 8) is the first of its kind and provides important evidence of effectiveness. The debate continues about appropriate methodology for the evaluation of health promotion initiatives and there have been important descriptive studies in the UK. The Barnet High Street Health Scheme was evaluated from the perspectives of pharmacist and consumer by Anderson and shown to have influenced community pharmacists' perceptions of their potential role in health promotion (Anderson, 1998a). The consumer evaluation of the scheme showed that those who had taken away leaflets from participating pharmacies were significantly more likely to be frequent visitors to the pharmacy, and to have one or more chronic illnesses (Anderson, 1998b). Anderson concluded that while those who are ill seek and value general health advice from pharmacists, assumptions about the extent to which healthy people might seek advice on health from pharmacies may have been ill-founded. Matheson similarly reports (Chapter 9) on community pharmacists contribution to the drug misuse problems and considers the perspective of both the professionals and the clients in this potentially controversial area of health promotion (Matheson, 1998).

Advice to other health professionals

The development of 'primary care pharmacists' has highlighted the pharmacist's role in advising general medical practitioners on prescribing issues at both policy and individual patient levels (Blenkinsopp *et al.*, 1998). This is an area where adoption following development has run ahead of formal validation through research and there have been few rigorous studies to assess effects, quality and outcomes. Descriptive studies without controls show that pharmacists make recommendations as a result of medication review and that these are adopted by general practitioners to varying degrees (see for example, Goldstein *et al.*, 1998). In a controlled trial Rodgers and colleagues (Rodgers *et al.*, 1999) demonstrated that pharmacist intervention in the general practice setting leads to reductions in prescribing costs. Tully and Cantrill's review of pharmacists' interventions concluded that they were consistently accompanied by improvements in clinical parameters (Tully and Cantrill, 1999), and a major randomised controlled trial of changes in clinical outcomes of hypertensive and angina patients after pharmacy review is ongoing (Fish *et al.*, 1999). Watson also demonstrated the positive benefit of using community pharmacists to deliver educational outreach evidence-based prescribing of NSAIDs to GPs (Watson, 2000).

Thus, the evidence base supporting the five key themes within Pharmacy in a New Age is growing but patchy. The remainder of this chapter will attempt to analyse key issues in moving forward.

The importance of research and development

Research and development, 'R & D', are often spoken of together. Yet in many cases in healthcare it has been difficult to see the links between them, and the NHS R & D programme has tended to focus on the 'R' at the expense of the 'D'. To take the analogy of a manufacturing enterprise, the job of researchers is to identify potential new products, while developers go on to test and refine potential products in the context of their future use. On the basis of this process, products are then developed to best fit the potential market.

One of the key issues in pharmacy practice has been the separation of these two processes. Development (the many pilot projects in service development for example) has suffered in two ways. Firstly too often it has not been based on previous research and secondly evaluation has generally not been rigorous. However, the findings of previous research can only be used where they exist and thus in a sense many pharmaceutical service development projects have been conducted in a relative vacuum. One of the important functions of this book is that it brings together important research and the 'state of the evidence' in relation to a range of roles for pharmacists.

The agenda for practitioners

Changes in the way healthcare is organised, delivered and commissioned offer many opportunities to pharmacists. The emphasis on evidence-based practice should be second nature to pharmacists, whose scientific training stresses the importance of evidence throughout. The emergence of clinical governance provides the basis not only for the application of evidence but also for monitoring and evaluation of outcomes.

Community pharmacists need to consider the evidence base for:

- the content of the information and advice that they give;
- the process by which that information is imparted.

Moreover, community pharmacists also need to consider these aspects not only for their own practice but also for that of their staff. Obvious starting points are:

- a formulary for OTC medicines;
- more documentation of recommended treatments, advice and referrals for both over-the-counter and prescribed medicines, and;
- improved mechanisms for feedback from patients so that outcomes can be recorded.

All of these will be needed if community pharmaceutical services such as prescribing on the NHS, or participating in funded services to provide advice on minor ailments are to be established. With the development of NHS Direct, the increasing use of protocols to provide a filter and decisions about referral is ongoing. NICE guidelines, disseminated through PRODIGY and more widely available, will cover minor ailments as well as chronic diseases. Potential purchasers of community pharmacy services will require robust systems for tracking the quality of service provided (including adherence to guidelines) and the outcomes achieved.

The agenda for researchers

As this book shows, pharmacy practice research has moved on considerably since Nicholas Mays' 1994 statement that it comprised 'small, descriptive feasibility studies, largely conducted by pharmacists'. Key indicators of progress have included:

- The development of multi-disciplinary research groups in Schools of Pharmacy (for example, the ground-breaking community pharmacy research conducted by the Manchester University team).
- The emergence of pharmacists as key players in other multi-disciplinary groups (for example Aberdeen University's Department of General Practice & Primary Care and London's School of Hygiene and Tropical Medicine.
- As a result, more research showing pharmacy in the wider context – management and user perspectives, for example, and more research using pluralistic methodological approaches.
- The publication of RPSGB's Pharmacy Practice Research Taskforce Report, demonstrating a more outward-looking Society forging closer links with key R & D organisations.
- The increasing quality, year on year, of papers presented at the health services research/pharmacy practice research conferences.
- The first outputs of the research consortium of funders (RPSGB, PSNC, major pharmacy employers). The development of this consortium illustrates the growing recognition of the importance of pharmacy practice research as a basis for evidence rather than an esoteric academic pursuit.
- Publication, through the Pharmacy Practice Research and Resource Centre, of research agendas on self-care and pharmacy, drug therapy and pharmacy, and workforce issues.
- Report of the Royal Pharmaceutical Society of Great Britain's Getting Research Into Practice working group, Medicines, Pharmacy and the NHS: Getting it right for patients and prescribers' (RPSGB, 1999).
- Fledgling community pharmacy research networks in Aberdeen, North Staffordshire, Southampton, Manchester and the Thames regions.

Nevertheless, again reflecting on Mays' critique, the next big step remains to 'explore what the profession as a whole can deliver and the relative costs and benefits of a service provided by the pharmacy profession in comparison to other health professionals'. The big questions around generalisability, feasibility across the range of community pharmacy settings, and cost-effectiveness in those settings, still remain. The repeat dispensing studies undertaken first in Scotland and more recently in England, and the smoking study reported in Chapter 8, offer the first move from research involving a small number of enthusiasts to all community pharmacists in particular areas. The establishment of community pharmacy research networks is promising and offers the opportunity for systematic study in the pharmacy setting.

The 1997 Cochrane Group review of the evidence of effectiveness of services provided by pharmacists struggled to source research studies of sufficient rigour to meet its criteria and identified a small number of such studies (Bero et al., 1997; Bero, 1998). The research agendas in medicines use and self-care have been identified and provide the basis for a more systematic and structured series of research programmes in pharmacy practice. Study designs can be further strengthened by even greater multi-disciplinary input to ensure that the standards of pharmacy practice research continue to improve. There is certainly a case for greater collaboration between groups of pharmacy practice researchers to mount multi-centre studies. There may also be a case for greater co-ordination of research to try to ensure that effort is not being duplicated and that key research questions are being addressed. The latter agenda has not even begun to be debated but pharmacy practice research needs to build on its strengths. Researchers may reject the notion that their agenda should be steered or guided but the benefits of collaboration and greater sharing of research plans could enrich pharmacy practice research and enhance its standing.

References

Anderson C (1998a). Health promotion by community pharmacists: perceptions, realities and constraints. *J Soc Admin Pharm* 15: 10–22.

Anderson C (1998b). Health promotion by community pharmacists: consumers' views. *Int J Pharm Pract* 6: 2–12.

Bero L A, Grilli R, Grimshaw J M (1998). Closing the gap between research and practice: an overview of systematic reviews of interventions to promote the implementation of research findings. *BMJ* 317: 465–68.

Bero L A, Mays N B, Bond C M, *et al.* (1997). Expanding pharmacists' roles and health services utilisation, costs and patient outcomes. *Cochrane Database of Reviews*.

Bissell P, Ward P R, Noyce P R (1997). Variation within community pharmacy (2): responding to the presentation of symptoms. *J Soc Admin Pharm* 14: 105–15.

Bissell P, Ward P R, Nogre P R (2000). Appropriateness measurement: application to advice-giving in community pharmacies. *Soc Sci Med* 51: 343–59.

Blenkinsopp A, Clarke W, Fisher M, *et al.* (1998). Implementing evidence in practice. In: Panton RS, Chapman S, eds. *Medicines management.* London: BMJ Books and Pharmaceutical Press.

Blenkinsopp A, Phelan M, Bourne J (2000). Extended adherence support by community pharmacists for patients with hypertension: a controlled trial. *Int J Pharm Pract* 8: in press.

Bond C M, Matheson C, Williams S, *et al.* (2000). Repeat Prescribing: a role for community pharmacists in monitoring and controlling repeat prescriptions. *Br J Gen Pract* 50: 271–5.

Coast-Senior E A, Kroner B A, Kelley C L, *et al.* (1998). Management of patients with type 2 diabetes by pharmacists in primary care clinics. *Ann Pharmacother* 32: 636–41.

Dowell J, Cruikshank J, Bain J, *et al.* (1998). Repeat dispensing by community pharmacists: advantages for patients and practitioners. *Br J Gen Pract* 48: 1858–9.

Fish A, Reid J, Bond C *et al.* (1999). Research project to evaluate the clinical outcomes of pharmacist attachments to practices in Grampian. In: *5th Health Service Research and Pharmacy Practice Conference, 1999,* Abstracts volume. Aston: Aston University.

Furniss L, Craig S K L, Scobie S, *et al.* (1998). Medication reviews in nursing homes: documenting and classifying the activities of a pharmacist. *Pharm J* 261: 320–3.

Goldstein R, Hulme H, Willits J (1998). Reviewing repeat prescribing – general practitioners and community pharmacists working together. *Int J Pharm Pract* 6: 60–6.

Gourley D R, Gourley G A, Solomon D K, *et al.* (1998a). Part 1. Development, implementation and evaluation of a multi-centre pharmaceutical care outcomes study. *J Am Pharm Assoc* 38: 567–73.

Gourley G A, Portner T S, Gourley D R, *et al.* (1998b). Part 3. Humanistic outcomes in the hypertension and COPD arms of a multi-centre outcomes study. *J Am Pharm Assoc* 38: 586–97.

Granas A G, Bates I (1999). The effect of pharmaceutical review of repeat prescriptions in general practice. *Int J Pharm Pract* 7: 264–74.

Mackie C A, Lauron D H, Campbell A, *et al.* (1999). A randomised controlled trial of medication review in patients receiving polypharmacy in a general practice setting. *Pharm J* Suppl. R7.

Matheson C (1998). Views of illicit drug users on their treatment and behaviour in Scottish community pharmacies: implications for harm reduction strategy. *Health Ed J* 57: 31–41.

McCombs J S, Liu G, Shi J, *et al.* (1998). The Kaiser Permanente/USC patient consultation study: change in use and cost of health care services. *Am J Health Syst Pharm* 55: 2485–89.

Rodgers S, Avery A J, Meechan D (1999). Controlled trial of pharmacists' intervention in general practice. *Br J Gen Pract* 49: 717–20.

Roins S, Benrimoj S I, Carroll P R, *et al.* (1998). Factors used by pharmacists in the recommendation of the active ingredient(s) and brand of non-prescription analgesics for a simple, tension and migraine headache. *Int J Pharm Pract* 6: 207–15.

Royal Pharmaceutical Society of Great Britain (1999). Medicines, pharmacy and the NHS: getting it right for patients and prescribers. *Report of the Getting Research into Practice Working Group*. London: Royal Pharmaceutical Society of Great Britain.

Solomon D K, Portner T S, Bass G E, *et al.* (1998). Part 2. Clinical and economic outcomes in the hypertension and COPD arms of a multi-centre outcomes study. *J Am Pharm Assoc* 38: 574–85.

Tully M P, Cantrill J (1999). Role of the pharmacist in evidence-based prescribing in primary care. In: Gabbay M, ed. *The Evidence-based Primary Care Handbook*. London: Royal Society of Medicine.

Ward P R, Bissell P, Noyce P R (1998). Medicines counter assistants: roles and responsibilities in the sale of deregulated medicines. *Int J Pharm Pract* 6: 207–15.

Watson M (2000). *Pharmaceutical Journal* (in press).

Index

Main discussions are indicated in **bold** type.